Life Goes On

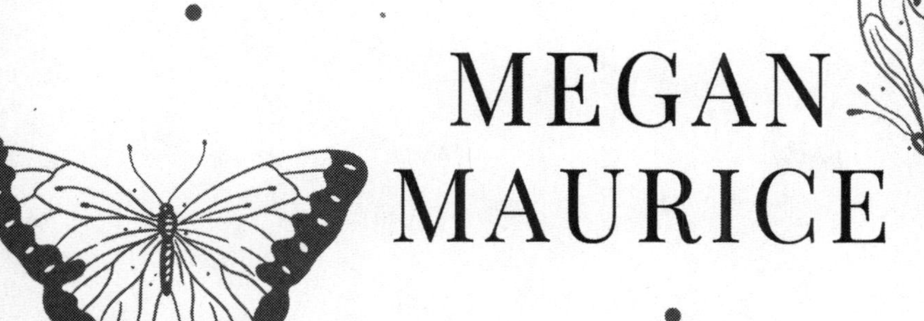

MEGAN
MAURICE

Life Goes On

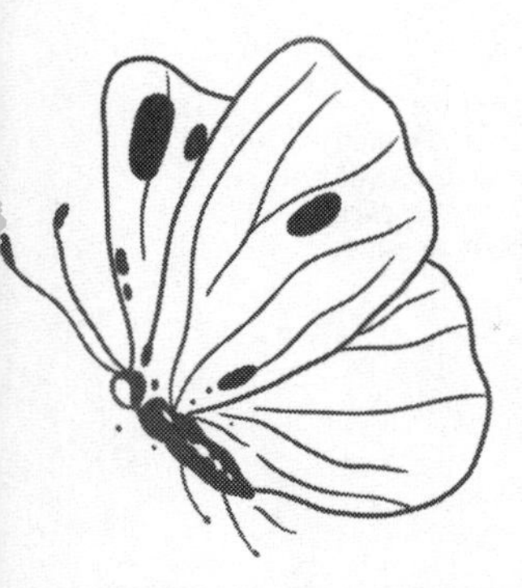

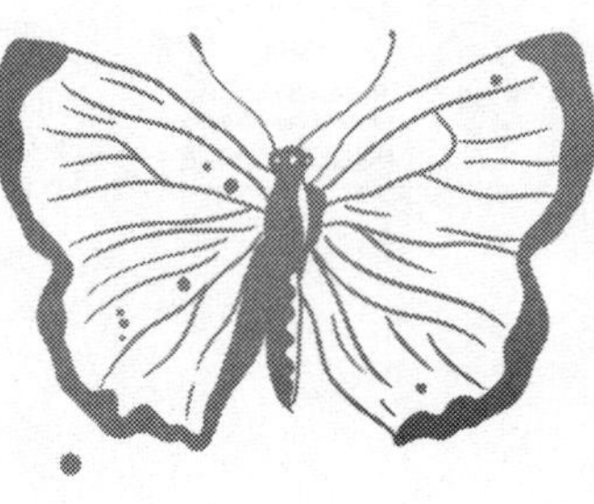

hachette
AUSTRALIA

This book contains references to sexual assault, suicide and domestic violence, which may be triggering for some readers. Discretion is advised.

hachette
AUSTRALIA

Published in Australia and New Zealand in 2024
by Hachette Australia
(an imprint of Hachette Australia Pty Limited)
Gadigal Country, Level 17, 207 Kent Street, Sydney, NSW 2000
www.hachette.com.au

Hachette Australia acknowledges and pays our respects to the past, present and future Traditional Owners and Custodians of Country throughout Australia and recognises the continuation of cultural, spiritual and educational practices of Aboriginal and Torres Strait Islander peoples. Our head office is located on the lands of the Gadigal people of the Eora Nation.

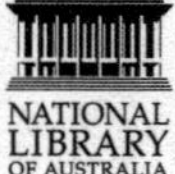

A catalogue record for this book is available from the National Library of Australia

ISBN: 978 0 7336 5086 4 (paperback)

Cover design and illustration by Louisa Maggio Design
Author photograph courtesy of Rhiannon Bertinshaw
Typeset in 12/18 pt Sabon LT Std by Kirby Jones
Printed and bound in Australia by McPherson's Printing Group

The paper this book is printed on is certified against the Forest Stewardship Council® Standards. McPherson's Printing Group holds FSC® chain of custody certification SA-COC-005379. FSC® promotes environmentally responsible, socially beneficial and economically viable management of the world's forests.

For my mum, Helen Maurice.

Thank you for all your research help,
and, more importantly, for always being there
for me and for making me who I am.

CONTENTS*

PROLOGUE Worst Day of My Life 1

CHAPTER ONE Waiting for My Real Life to Begin 9

CHAPTER TWO The Wolves 35

CHAPTER THREE Bury Me Deep in Love 63

CHAPTER FOUR I Won't Let You Go 85

CHAPTER FIVE Like I Used To 115

CHAPTER SIX You're the Voice 143

CHAPTER SEVEN Linger 177

CHAPTER EIGHT Leaps and Bounds 205

CHAPTER NINE Sunshine on a Rainy Day 233

CHAPTER TEN I Am Here 263

REFERENCES 283

ACKNOWLEDGEMENTS 291

---

* Author's note: When I started chemotherapy, I wasn't allowed to have any visitors with me in the hospital due to Covid protocols. I asked my friends and family to each add one song to a playlist that I could listen to during my chemo sessions – something that would remind me of them or make me feel less alone in some way. The chapter titles of this book have all been drawn from that playlist.

PROLOGUE

Worst Day of My Life

After my third chemotherapy session, I thought I knew what to expect. I knew about the nausea and fatigue. I'd made it through mouth sores, cracked lips and painful swallowing. I'd discovered the very annoying need to 'listen to my body' and not just push through, hoping the side effects would go away. But my god, I wanted to make it to a long-awaited holiday.

Originally planned for July 2021, Covid lockdowns had forced us to move it to January, where it fell five days after my third chemo session. We weren't going far – it was less than an hour away. During that time of lockdowns and border closures, holidays close to home seemed like the safest option.

I had been cleared by my oncologists to travel, as long as I promised to research where the nearest emergency department was and take a thermometer and my little 'please let me into your hospital quickly, I have cancer' card with me so I could rush off if my temperature hit 38 degrees. Still, we didn't dare to believe it might really happen. No-one allowed themselves to get excited until we actually arrived at our destination. At any moment, a complication in my illness or one of us being identified as a close contact of someone with Covid could swiftly shut the whole thing down.

But finally, the day was here and everyone was okay. Against my better judgement, I pushed through the fatigue and nausea to get everything ready. My daughter, Pia, and I bundled up our cats and took them to my parents' house. I tried – and failed – to convince my mum that I was totally fine as I rested on her couch before I could face getting back in the car. She took my blood pressure and looked at me in only the way a parent of an adult making an ill-informed decision can as I smiled through the pain and left the house.

With everything packed, Pia and I headed to my husband Shaun's work to pick him up and get straight on the road. Relieved of driving responsibilities, I started to crumble immediately. I needed to lie down, but I had to keep sitting, push through a little bit longer. When we arrived, it took what felt like years to find the disorganised accommodation manager and be let into our cabin.

With blackness closing in around me, I stumbled inside and straight into bed. For three days of our week-long holiday, I barely left it. While the fatigue and nausea were close to unbearable, the guilt was possibly even worse. I had made it to this holiday to spend precious time with my family and I couldn't even drag myself out of bed.

Chemo fatigue is like nothing I have ever experienced. It's not simply the inability to get out of bed. For those three days, I couldn't watch TV, look at social media, read a book or even listen to music or a podcast. Any attempt to pass the time in any vaguely interesting way left me feeling even more wretched. Nor could I sleep properly. At night, I managed to doze on and off, but during the day, I felt too sick and there was nothing I could do but stare at the ceiling and wonder when it would end.

Eventually, the side effects subsided. I emerged from bed, and the remaining time we spent there was lovely. I was slowly able to recover from my guilt of having missed such a big chunk of the trip, but those three days are burnt into my brain as some of the most traumatic of my illness. Over a year on, I can feel the tension in my body rising as I recount the details.

While those intense periods after each chemo session were incredibly awful, throughout the rest of my cancer treatment and beyond, I felt numb. I was diagnosed with breast cancer at thirty-six years old. Up until that point, I had been the picture of health and had no family history of the illness. My diagnosis came suddenly – wildly out of the blue – and turned my life upside down. Only it felt like I turned upside down as well; there I was, walking normally on the ceiling and wondering why everyone was looking at me. I adjusted so quickly to this new upside-down life, I often found myself comforting others who were upset by my diagnosis. In the absence of any other ideas or feelings, I made myself a 'positive attitude' mask and wore it every day, posting about my experiences on social media and feeling surprised when people said I was 'strong' or 'brave'. I didn't feel either. I felt like I was playing a character in a sad-but-uplifting show, and all I knew was that it was very important to keep playing this part and see this through to the end.

When the end of treatment came, I felt sure the feelings would come with it. I would unstick myself from the ceiling, crumple to the floor, remove my mask and finally process this whole confusing riddle. But the time never came. As I watched the 'cancer patient' persona slip off my shoulders, I kept coming back to a quote I remembered reading as a teenager: 'In three words I can sum up everything I've learned about life. It goes on.'

These words – attributed to American poet Robert Frost in 1954 – have stayed hidden in the recesses of my mind for many years, but suddenly they hurtled their way to the front as the only real knowledge I could find to explain what it is like to live after such a life-changing and traumatic event.

I started to understand that I needed to somehow get myself to my 'it goes on' point. It was clear that it wasn't going to happen on its own, and equally clear that I couldn't just go back to living the same life as before I had cancer. I felt like I was returning home to a place that belonged to someone I didn't quite remember being. And so I started to search for ideas and pieces of wisdom that could guide me to the place where my life could start to make sense again.

The more I thought about what this place might look like for me, the more curious I became about others who had managed to find their own. As much as the self-centred voice in my head might like to believe I was the first person in the world to encounter trauma and come out the other side, there are millions of other people in the world who have gone through this. No-one's trauma is quite the same and no-one's recovery is either. But by starting conversations and beginning to stitch all these experiences and responses together, I am hoping to combine and create something that feels like my way to go on in the world. To do so, I know I need to encounter trauma in all its forms. To explore the knowledge of only those who have recovered from breast cancer, or even cancer in general, would be failing to understand the bigger picture. What I am struggling to understand, to cope with, is the trauma that cancer left me with; the illness was simply its vessel.

I wanted to write down the wisdom that I've gained because I know there are so many people out there who have felt, or will one day feel what I am feeling. Like you're building a life from scratch and you have absolutely nothing to go on. Maybe you will find some healing and an idea of your way forward in these pages.

I never imagined on that awful day in the depths of chemo sickness that I would have any worries when this was all over. I thought making it out of that body that didn't feel like mine would propel me into the new life I needed to have. Instead, it left me confused – transported into yet another body that doesn't feel like mine, one that is numb and still barely stumbling through the world.

In Gail Honeyman's novel *Eleanor Oliphant is Completely Fine*, the protagonist is living a life marred by trauma that she has not yet processed. Once she finally comes to terms with it, she tells her concerned friend, 'In the end, what matters is this: I survived.'

It is a logical place to arrive at after living through a traumatic event, but it is one that I find little comfort in. There must be more to this than survival. And I am determined to find out what it is.

CHAPTER ONE

Waiting for My Real Life to Begin

Well, here we are. Today I had my final radiation. It's kind of a strange bit of treatment to finish on, because it's so non-invasive – it doesn't feel like a huge moment the way finishing chemo did. Though the feeling of going in every weekday will definitely stay with me – I'm sure I'll have a little internal panic at 1pm every day thinking I need to leave the house!

This isn't completely the end of treatment. It's just – as my friend Kylie so eloquently put it – the point where being a cancer patient stops being my full-time job. I'll have annual scans for the rest of my life, plus annual follow-ups with my surgeon, medical oncologist and radiation oncologist for the next five years.

In a couple of weeks, I start hormone therapy, which involves a daily tablet and a monthly injection to put me into menopause. My cancer is oestrogen and progesterone positive, so it's important to stop my body producing these hormones so the cancer doesn't have anything to feed off and regrow. That treatment will last five to ten years.

So relatively speaking, I'm very early on in my treatment journey. But I like to think this first part was the really precarious, rocky, hilly part of the road and now I'm just up to the part that's very long and boring and you wish it was over, but at least it's flat and free of too many obstacles.

I'm sure I'll have more thoughts and feelings once this whole experience actually hits me one day – it still feels a bit like it's happening to someone else and I'm watching it all. But for now, I'm just very grateful that I no longer have to drive up and down Parramatta Road every day.

These are the words I wrote on social media after my cancer treatment finished.

I committed to charting my progress, but when I sat down to put together that final update, I felt lost for words.

It wasn't that I thought people were particularly hanging out to find out my thoughts, but I had been using my social media posts as a diary of sorts – the kind that provides little serotonin boosts when people like or comment – so I had more incentive to keep it going, which I absolutely would not have if I'd just written my thoughts down privately in a notebook.

But for this last one, I wanted some powerful and meaningful words for myself so that down the track when I scroll back through my timeline, there will be a little snapshot of this moment in time which captures what I am thinking and feeling. The problem is, I'm not thinking or feeling anything. Truly, the only thing that I can hold on to at all is the relief of not having to get in my car every day and freedom from panic that delays in being seen at the clinic would make me late to school pick-up. How peculiar to reach this moment which felt like it should be incredibly climactic and significant and instead be caught up in the mundane.

I don't know what exactly I expected. I thought it would be more than minor concerns about what time I arrived at school in the afternoons. I don't think I needed it to be an epiphany or even for the emotions that hit me to be positive. From the moment of my diagnosis in October 2021, I had been waiting for the full mental breakdown to hit me. When it became clear that I was going to continue to coast along in what one friend who was also going through cancer treatment referred to as 'survival mode', I eventually began to think of it as a similar experience to running a marathon.

I have run exactly one marathon in my life, and I remember it so vividly that I simply was not able to convince myself to do another one. The thing about running a marathon is that you absolutely cannot think about what you're doing while you're doing it. You don't train the full distance beforehand because if your body knew what you were up to, it would just refuse to go on. You have to sneak up on it, run thirty-five kilometres a week or two before the race and then taper down, pretend that you're done with all that silly long-distance and you're about to get back to more sensible things. And then – BAM – you hit it with 42.2 kilometres when it's least expecting it.

I assumed that subconsciously I had gone into this mode – pushing through with my head down, not allowing any emotions in lest I found myself crying by the roadside and asking passers-by to carry me to the finish line. This made sense. I just had to prepare myself for the emotions to hit me all at the end. When I finished my *actual* marathon, I stumbled through the finish chute and collected my medal and finishers' t-shirt. I found a volunteer and asked for directions to the area of the recovery village where I'd agreed to meet my dad and my husband. He pointed up a hill, and I sat down and sobbed my heart out, so colossal did that small hill seem in my post-marathon state. While I'd rather not have had an embarrassing emotional breakdown in front of this unfortunate volunteer, it was at least a reaction that made sense to me; I had put my body through something incredibly hard and now it was over and I was processing it.

I prime myself so many times for the emotional outburst to happen. Will it be when I am interviewing a cancer researcher for work? That would be embarrassing, but at least she'd be understanding. Will it be during my twelve-month scan? Again, not the worst place for it, it's probably something they've seen a few times before. Or will it happen completely randomly? Will I collapse to the ground in tears when I'm paying for my groceries or catching the train to work? I am prepared for any and all of it. What I am not prepared for is for it not happening at all. Feeling stuck, like I'm permanently in a numb state was the last thing I expected, and I have no idea how to deal with it. I don't even cry during sad moments on television shows like I used to.

While I'm not necessarily hoping to have a mental breakdown, it feels like something that has to happen before I can move on. Is it the lack of a meltdown that is responsible for the limbo that I feel stuck in? I start to believe if I had a better understanding of trauma and how it manifests in the mind and body, I could figure out what has happened to me and find a way to recover.

It took me a while to even accept that what I have been through is trauma. I don't feel like that word belongs to me – it is the domain of people who have been in terrifying accidents or suffered through unthinkable abuse. It seems like something that happens all at once and unexpectedly, something that has a clear moment where you know something terrible is happening. What I experienced was instead a slow unravelling of everything I knew, with no moment of clarity. Could that really be trauma? I seek out information and definitions, which reiterate that trauma comes as a result of events that threaten our safety – such as abuse, life-threatening illness, being in close proximity to natural disasters, being a victim of a crime, the death of someone close or being in an accident.[1] While cancer undoubtedly counts as a life-threatening illness, I still struggle to place my experiences in that box.

But one point that I keep reading in multiple books and articles stands out to me – highly emotional reactions to trauma are normal and, for most people, the effects subside within days or weeks. I find that intriguing; that so many people encounter these life-changing experiences, process them and move on. According to the data, a very small minority of people develop conditions such as post-traumatic stress disorder (PTSD), the rate of the disorder in the general population is reportedly between 1.3 per cent and 8.3 per cent.[2] I was curious to know if this could be underreported – perhaps people suffering from the aftereffects of trauma are unable to access the kind of mental health care needed to make this diagnosis? Or perhaps some have not realised the significance of their symptoms and thus have not sought a diagnosis.

Or maybe it's just that PTSD is only one reaction to trauma and the fact that it sits at the extreme end of the scale is what makes it so notable. But just because someone isn't suffering from PTSD doesn't mean they have fully processed their trauma and are able to live a 'normal' life again. How many people are sitting somewhere in between those two extremes, unable to return to the life they knew before, but not so far away from it that they are unable to function?

Trauma as something related to the mental and emotional states of being is a relatively new idea. The word comes from the Greek *traumatikos*, meaning 'wound', and was originally used in medical science to exclusively mean a severe physical injury. It took on the connection to psychological injury following the Vietnam War and the diagnosis of PTSD was added to the Diagnostic and Statistical Manual of Mental Disorders in 1980.[3] Even once trauma was recognised as a psychological condition, the belief remained that it was only experienced by soldiers who had fought in wars. Psychiatrist Judith Herman widened the definition after discovering similar symptoms in women who had experienced sexual abuse.[4] From there, the theory around trauma continued to expand to encompass a wider range of experiences.

Trauma theory scholar Meera Atkinson says trauma develops 'when the psyche fails to register and process an experience because it happens too fast or too forcefully, overwhelming the thinking brain and the nervous system.'[5] She explains that while most people who experience harrowing events suffer from stress and distress, which are similar to trauma in the way they present in the body, the key difference is that trauma actually changes the way the brain functions. While stress and distress occur at the time of the event and can linger for a short time afterward, trauma keeps the brain in a state of constant hypervigilance. The emotional symptoms stay at the same level long after the event is over. In short, where trauma exists, the brain does not understand that the danger is over.

PTSD is the disorder most commonly associated with trauma, but it is only one of the responses that may be triggered. Dissociative identity disorder (DID, formerly known as multiple personality disorder) is one such response to childhood trauma, when a child's 'psychological development is disrupted by early repetitive trauma that prevents the normal processes of consolidating a core sense of identity.'[6] Essentially, young people affected by repeated trauma develop multiple states of being – sometimes designed to cope with specific situations. People who are exposed to a traumatic event commonly develop acute stress disorder (ASD), which has similar symptoms to PTSD, but these only occur in the short term, usually resolving less than a month after the incident that triggered them. People can be initially diagnosed with ASD and go on to be diagnosed with PTSD if symptoms do not resolve.[7]

So pronounced are the biological effects of trauma that work is being done into developing a blood test that could diagnose PTSD. A study on war veterans was able to identify particular genetic markers that underwent the biggest changes during high stress situations. The discovery of these markers could also play a part in better developing treatments for PTSD and provide the opportunity to individualise treatments based on the specific genetic markers of a person.[8] The findings are still quite new and there will undoubtedly be more work done to understand what they mean and how such a blood test could be carried out in the general population. But it is nonetheless interesting to consider the physiological impacts that trauma has and the way it changes the landscape of the brain and the body in such a deliberate way. Research has shown that there are similarities between a brain affected by PTSD and one that has suffered from mild traumatic brain injury, with ongoing changes to connectivity and emotional regulation common to both afflictions.[9] My reading also uncovers the answer to a question I have pondered from the start, as I find research suggesting that PTSD is extremely underdiagnosed.[10] It is likely then that many people do not realise the way their body and brain has been altered by trauma, and as such are not finding effective treatments but are simply trying to go on as best they can.

It is a complex landscape, unsurprisingly given that trauma itself is so complex and takes in all manner of different experiences and reactions. It makes me realise just how misunderstood trauma and its associated conditions are – I think of the many times I heard people claiming to be suffering from PTSD due to lockdowns during the pandemic. While these were undoubtedly times of great stress for a lot of people, particularly those who lived alone and people with young children, it is unlikely that many of those people are still in a state of heightened anxiety with a brain that does not understand that lockdown has ended, or altered gene expression making permanent changes to their bodies. While PTSD from lockdown could certainly have developed for people in volatile situations, like violent relationships and insecure housing, the vast majority of people likely experienced stress rather than trauma.

Having this distinction in my mind helps me to feel more comfortable with labelling what I experienced as trauma, even if I am not sure what I am experiencing now is PTSD. For although my overwhelming feelings have been numbness and a sense that this was somehow not real, there is a strong belief deep within me that I am not safe and that this is not over. I feel irrevocably changed by my experience and I struggle to believe that there are no cancer cells lurking within me, just waiting to make themselves known. My unexpected diagnosis shook me to my very core and has taken away from me a sense of safety and faith that things will work out in the end.

I remember the first time I suffered a moderately serious injury playing sport, where I tore some of the ligaments in my ankle. I have never again played with the freedom I did before that injury, because from that point, I truly carried with me the knowledge that things could go wrong.

It was no longer an abstract idea: something that happened to other people but not to me. The awareness weighed heavily on me. Now with the life-and-death ramifications of cancer, that weight is even more burdensome.

The numbness itself is also an interesting symptom. While I have taken it as a signifier that what I went through may not have been trauma – because I'm not having episodes involving highly emotional flashbacks – I discover that emotional numbness is a fairly common trauma response. In fact, there has been significant research to demonstrate that emotional numbness is often linked to more severe PTSD and a weaker response to psychological treatment.[11]

The numbness I felt during my 'survival mode' was likely a form of dissociation – a common and normal response to trauma that protects the body and brain from being overwhelmed. It is the 'freeze' component of the 'flight, fight or freeze' response, cutting off contact between the brain and body in order to get through what is happening.[12] It is a response I associate with the kind of trauma that is acute and happening in the moment – trauma that involves a violent act. It makes sense to me that dissociation would happen in those circumstances because of the presence of a physical threat. I haven't connected it with my experience because the threat is so abstract and slow-moving. It doesn't seem like something I can dissociate from, but from discussions with the psychologist at the cancer hospital and reading studies, I have a better understanding of what my brain was doing to survive. Only now I feel stuck, unsure how to let my brain know that the danger has passed.

It is difficult to rid myself of this response in part because there is no guarantee I am safe. Many of the therapies used for people who have suffered trauma start with a first step of establishing safety and trying to do exactly what I wish I could – teach the trauma-altered brain that the danger has passed. While that is the case for me – my treatment was successful in eliminating the cancer from my body – a key attribute of cancer is that it sometimes comes back. So while I am out of the war zone, it feels like I could be suddenly returned there at any time. As such, the hypervigilance is hard to shake. It is something I still need to learn how to do.

In recent years, there have been more discussions and a greater understanding of cancer as a form of trauma. Research has found that over twenty per cent of cancer patients develop PTSD within the first six months of diagnosis[13] – a rate similar to soldiers returning from war. Researchers note that although PTSD is highly prevalent in cancer communities, it is not well understood or treated, in part due to outdated notions of trauma (like I held) being related to acute physical threats. As well as this, cancer patients often feel the need to be strong and positive or adopt a 'warrior mentality', leading to them refusing to admit that they are not coping and thus not seeking treatment.[14] While for many people, PTSD symptoms decrease over time – the 2018 study found that the twenty per cent experiencing symptoms at the six-month mark dropped to six per cent by four years following diagnosis – many of those whose symptoms remain experience a worsening of their PTSD over the years.

Research has also delved into the specific connection between breast cancer and PTSD, with some environmental and biological risk factors being identified. The more advanced and aggressive the cancer, the higher the risk of developing PTSD, and women under fifty have also been found to be more likely to experience PTSD symptoms. Researchers suggest too that anti-endocrine therapies (medications that block oestrogen and progesterone in patients with hormone receptor positive breast cancers, like mine) may interrupt activation of the amygdala – the region of the brain responsible for processing emotions. This in turn can lead to altered reactions to threat stimuli, which some scientists believe could be linked to the development of PTSD.[15]

What this can look like is having extreme reactions to relatively straightforward situations – for example, having panic attacks in medical settings, even when the appointment is not related to cancer. The altered brain automatically sees that environment as a threat and is not able to distinguish between the trauma encountered in that setting previously and its different meaning in the present time.

Anti-endocrine therapies, such as tamoxifen, the drug I am taking, are known to be correlated with mental health issues such as anxiety and depression. This is possibly due to the role of one type of oestrogen in modulating serotonin receptors, which regulate mood.[15] It may explain some of the difficulties breast cancer patients face in trying to return to a normal life after the trauma of diagnosis and treatment. It is a never-ending wave of symptoms and challenges that completely alter our perception of normal and leave us adrift of our former selves.

In my experience, issues like this are less commonly discussed with breast cancer patients, because these anti-endocrine therapies are very effective at preventing cancer recurrence, which is the first and most important goal of oncologists. The ongoing impact on quality of life for the patients seems to be a secondary concern. This is not the fault of individual oncologists who are doing everything in their power to keep their patients alive and offering the best treatments available. Rather it is reflective of a black and white medical system that sees simply the preservation of life as a success, with no room for the shades of grey that make up the quality of that life.

The more that as we as a society begin to understand about trauma, the more we are finding its roots buried everywhere we look. It is something that is likely to grow beneath all of us at one point or another in our lifetimes. For some communities, it is woven into the fabric of their being. Australia's First Nations people experience trauma at a disproportionately high level due to the ongoing effects of colonisation on the world's oldest continuing culture. In her book, *Trauma Trails, Recreating Song Lines: The Transgenerational Effects of Trauma in Indigenous Australia*, Jiman and Bundjalung woman Judy Atkinson explores the different kinds of trauma that First Nations communities experience and offers a road to healing. Atkinson looks at the ramifications of collective trauma, which she notes often has enduring effects on an entire population. 'It seeps slowly and insidiously into the fabric and soul of relations and beliefs of people as a community,' she writes. 'The shock of loss of self and community comes gradually. People, feeling bereaved, grieve for their loss of cultural surrounds, as well as for family and friends.'[16]

Collective and intergenerational trauma are incredibly

complex, tied up in the biological effects of trauma on the body that are then coded into DNA and passed down to children and grandchildren. This occurs when 'the effects of a traumatic event or issue are passed down through generations via genes, biology and then through environments that exist as threatening to oneself, such as racism.'[17] The longer trauma continues, the more likely it is to be passed down. It is overwhelming to think about how many lives have been touched by trauma and how many more will be in the future, whether directly or indirectly. Its reach cannot be underestimated.

Despite the greater understanding of trauma that has begun to be developed and advances in neuroscience, there has been little change to the process of diagnosing and treating people suffering from PTSD and other trauma-related conditions. One study suggests this is partly due to disagreement within the field about the definition of the disorders themselves and examines the possibility of focusing on the core dimensions of some of the most prominent symptoms in order to create a treatment plan for those, rather than getting caught up in the diagnosis.[18] Whether or not clinicians agree on if someone meets the criteria for PTSD, the symptoms can be treated and managed in the best way to help the person experiencing them move on with life. In this study, researchers focused on one of the most disruptive symptoms of PTSD – intrusive traumatic reexperiencing. People who report this symptom 'involuntarily and vividly relive the traumatic event' in different forms, including nightmares and flashbacks.[19] Although I do not experience this particular symptom, I am interested in the idea of focusing on the symptoms rather than the diagnosis. Of all the people I have spoken to who have experienced traumatic events, only a handful have been diagnosed with PTSD, but all of them have endured the effects of trauma in different ways and have witnessed their lives and bodies become marked and changed through symptoms. Shifting the dial toward understanding those symptoms and how people are affected by them – regardless of their diagnosis – seems more likely to help people move on with their lives.

In considering trauma and the reverberations it creates in a life and a body, my mind continually turns back to Bri Lee's haunting memoir *Eggshell Skull.* In this groundbreaking book, Lee details her experiences as a judge's associate, working primarily on cases dealing with child sexual abuse. It is an incredibly beautifully written, heartbreaking book and one that has stayed with me since the moment I finished reading it.

The book feels like two stories – one the recounting of Lee's year as a judge's associate, the stories of the trials she works on, her frustrations at the shortcomings of the legal system, the difficult world that she has immersed herself in. The second is a slow unravelling of the person who stepped into this world as each day she is forced to reckon with her own trauma amid constant reminders. This second story is like a jigsaw puzzle, with pieces scattered throughout the first, allowing the reader to collect and assemble them as they bear witness to Lee's disentanglement from herself.

Lee describes the feeling of living with the memory that is slowly destroying her: 'I read once that the human body slowly pushes shrapnel back out through the skin,' she writes. 'That a shard of metal can take years to reach the surface and finally, truly be expelled. Could the same thing happen to memories? Perhaps that was what I was feeling: an itchy, irksome thing, a foreign object inside me, moving just millimetres every year, tearing through me until it breached.'[20]

There is a vividness to this imagery that calls to me so loudly, that has stayed niggling away in the back of my mind in the years since I first read the book and returns to me when I begin considering my experience as taking place in the realms of trauma. The physical presence of trauma within the body, slowly pushing its way to the surface and no longer allowing itself to be ignored, is something I feel deeply – so much so that I can almost feel it moving, wriggling its way closer and closer to my skin.

The months of my recovery tick on and the emotional breakdown I feel sure is coming continues to stay away, so I begin to look for other ways to heal. No longer treading so cautiously with the expectation of floods of tears enveloping me when I least expect it, I begin searching for answers in other places. I start by seeing a psychologist provided by the cancer centre I am being treated in. Just in case you're thinking 'women will literally write an entire book about how they haven't recovered from their trauma instead of going to therapy', I do go to therapy. The psychologist is excellent – she is kind and listens intently to what I say and gently offers up alternatives when I find myself stuck in the rigid ruts of my preconceived ideas. But there are so many aspects of my experience that I don't feel like I can explain, or that she could understand. Her consistent reassurances that 'survival mode' is a good and valid way of dealing with a traumatic experience help. At the same time, she feels that this response also means I have processed my emotions and should be able to move on, while I fundamentally feel that I have not. I truly appreciate her perspective and I consider it seriously, but it was a point of disagreement that we cannot reconcile. I walk away feeling like I need something more.

During this time of treatment and recovery, I also have been finding myself having more and more conversations with people in my life who have experienced different kinds of trauma. Some are people I know well, others are at the periphery of my life or their paths intersect with mine by chance. I realise that I want to record these stories. Ever since I was very young, writing has helped me make meaning from the world around me. Each person I talk to has a unique perspective and I feel that writing down what I learn will help me understand it and maybe start to apply it to my own life.

Some of the conversations I have are complete stories told within these pages, while others have left their echoes in my understanding of trauma and the way I am telling my own story. I want to share these experiences because hearing these stories and understanding people's lives makes me feel less alone.

When I first start talking to people more purposefully, many friends and family members express concern for my mental health and want to make sure I have support in place to help protect myself before opening myself up to other people's trauma. I heed their warnings and speak about my idea with the psychologist, who is able to be my safety net if I need support throughout the process of talking and writing. At first, I also try to focus the conversations around people's recovery from trauma rather than the traumatic event itself. This is something I think will help both me and the people I am talking to. I am wary of upsetting them, of opening up old wounds, by talking about these dark times. But the more I talk, the more I realise that many people are open to speaking about their trauma. By approaching these conversations sensitively and with a genuine interest in the people I am talking to and their feelings, I find that very little is off-limits. In fact, many people welcome the opportunity to talk openly and honestly about their darkest times. It makes me realise how often in our culture we say nothing out of fear of saying the wrong thing and how much better we can be at softly addressing tragedy in the lives of those around us.

It is something I wish I had understood better in the past – I know that I have avoided bringing up subjects with friends or have been guilty of responding with something bordering on toxic positivity due to my own unease with the situation. It is not something I understood consciously as I unravelled these long-held notions of how to speak about uncomfortable topics, it happened little by little during my conversations with people who had recovered from trauma. It is only now that I am reflecting on it that I understand the importance of breaking down those barriers and acknowledging – and even embracing – the messiness of people's lives.

In *A Heart That Works*, Rob Delaney delves into the heartbreaking experience of his two-year-old son dying of brain cancer. It is a book that covers the full spectrum of emotions, from joy to devastation. In one part, he reflects on his feelings when he tells one of his son's carers that the cancer has returned after a period of remission. The carer yells and cries at the horror of it and Delaney is surprisingly heartened by this response. 'She recoiled from the news as if I'd hit her,' he writes. 'Her response was like water in the desert for me ... it beat the hell out of a lot of the English and American responses (we) were getting from people when they heard the news ... In the years since I think of it often as the best response I received. It helped me.'[21]

I think about myself, about Rob Delaney and about everyone I have spoken to in the course of writing this book. It feels like we are living in a slightly different world to those around us. We can talk to the people in that other world, but those conversations are never going to be the same as the ones we have in our own trauma-altered one. The people on the other side can love and care for us unendingly, they can turn their lives upside down to help us, but they can never fully understand the experience and as such may always find it hard to say the 'right' thing.

When I first shared my diagnosis, I was bombarded with love, offers of assistance and gifts. Most people's responses fell into the categories of 'you've got this', 'sending healing vibes' or 'you're so strong/brave'. But one friend who had been through her own breast cancer diagnosis some years earlier sent me a message saying that she was devastated by the news and that she cried and screamed for me when she found out. Like Delaney, I find this kind of response so much more heartening. I hold no ill-regard for those who sent positive and uplifting messages – I had been framing everything I wrote about my diagnosis so positively, so it was unsurprising to see this reflected back to me. But it wasn't until I received this different kind of response that I realised how much I had craved it. Something awful was happening to me and I felt validated by her recognition.

I find that speaking to other people about their trauma is far from difficult for me; it is actually comforting and healing. Knowing that I am not alone in the ways I am struggling helps a lot, as does listening to people unpack their feelings and put their deepest fears into words. The conversations are rambling, tear-stained and full of emotion and heart. I try to listen much more than I talk and make it clear that I don't expect anyone to talk about anything they're not comfortable with. Over the months and years, I collect stories and extract wisdom and lessons from within them. No two experiences with trauma are the same, but there are common threads that link them, winding their way from one person to the next and telling a story of their own in the journey.

Each of the chapters that follow is shaped around a theme that has been vital to my recovery and the wisdom I received from the people who spoke to me. From managing fear and worry, to parenting, friendship, work, advocacy, coping with ongoing impacts of trauma, being active and creating a new life from the wreckage of trauma, each of these subjects carries weight for me as something I need to resolve before I truly feel able to move on.

Each person's story contains many different ideas and pieces of wisdom that have helped me start to articulate my own story and understand how it evolves. But as I speak and write and put these stories together, I feel that each of the nine people whose stories are shared within these pages leaves me with a significant insight into a particular aspect of life after trauma.

In order to dig myself out of these ruts I have found myself stuck in, I need to get my head around these areas of my life and understand how the pieces of me fit together. It is a daunting task and one I am not sure I have the strength and courage to take on. But the alternative feels like a nonexistence, a between place without real feelings or experiences. If I want to move forward rather than this perpetual sideways motion, I need to confront the unknown and do the work to understand how to go on.

CHAPTER TWO

The Wolves

'You learn how to manage pain in your life through painful events.'

When I think about the possibility of my cancer returning, one image repeats itself over and over. It is from *Catching Fire*, the second book in Suzanne Collins's *Hunger Games* trilogy. The protagonist – Katniss Everdeen – has just discovered that she will be sent into the Hunger Games arena to fight to the death for the second time. It is much worse than before because now she truly understands the horrors that await her. On hearing the news, Katniss runs blindly from her home, with no plans of where she is going, only knowing that she has to run away from the news. When she eventually stops, she stuffs the front of her shirt into her mouth and screams until her voice is gone.

I can't imagine any other reaction to the news that I am about to face the same trauma again. Deep down, I have this feeling of entitlement to a life free from terrible things – I did the hard thing and it's over now. That was the deal. It's unfair to make me go through it again. It's childish reasoning, but it's something I think most people deeply and inexplicably believe. Unfortunately, one of the biggest risk factors for getting cancer is having had cancer before. Whether that is a secondary cancer developing as a result of treatment not being effective in eliminating all the cancer cells, or a second primary cancer that may be caused by the treatments (such as chemotherapy or radiotherapy) for the first primary cancer, it is something that plays on the minds of many cancer survivors.

The official name of this series of worries that I find myself entangled in is a 'fear of recurrence'. I can't speak for every cancer survivor, but for me what makes this fear so acute is that I would be walking in with my eyes open. The first time around it was like walking into a forest in the darkest part of the night. I could imagine the horrors that lay in wait around every corner, but I didn't know for sure they were there and there was every chance I would walk out the other side relatively unscathed. Being diagnosed a second time would feel like being dragged, kicking and screaming, back to the same forest in broad daylight, with the thorny path exposed and unavoidable, the wolves in plain sight. We often talk about 'fear of the unknown' and 'better the devil you know' but when you have been pushed to your limits and faced pain like you have never known before, the unknown starts to seem a lot more palatable.

I've come to understand that I'm probably never going to move on from this fear. I can make it take up less space in my life, make it manageable, but it will always be with me. My fears became more acute during my recovery when the stories of Olivia Newton-John and Maria Cummins (mother of Australian men's cricket captain Pat Cummins) hit the media. Both women were diagnosed with breast cancer at a relatively young age, while parenting young children. They endured treatment and recovered only to have a recurrence many years down the track that eventually killed them. While the majority of cancers have the highest risk of recurrence within the first five years of the initial diagnosis, in oestrogen-receptor-positive breast cancer approximately fifty per cent of recurrences happen outside of that five-year period.[22]

Hearing those stories makes the possibility of cancer recurrence a lot more real. Newton-John's initial diagnosis was in 1992 and her recurrence happened over twenty years later, while Cummins was diagnosed in 2006 and died in 2023. Although an extra twenty years of life after cancer is not to be taken lightly, I know that I can never accept that as my fate. I cannot feel at peace with the belief that cancer will inevitably come back for me.

In trying to learn more about my fear of recurrence, I discover some academic research that has led to the creation of a system for oncologist-led interventions to address these fears with patients.[23] The idea is that patients already have a relationship with their oncologist, which will assist in normalising their fears and personalising the experience. It also allows patients to get assistance within the existing structures of follow-up appointments rather than requiring separate sessions with breast care nurses or psychologists.

I read the journal articles produced from this study with great interest and with my own follow-up appointment approaching, I tuck the idea into my back pocket. I meet with my oncologist and we speak about the side effects from the medications I am taking and how to manage them. At last, she broaches the topic I want to talk about.

'Do you ever worry about the cancer coming back?' she asks me.

'Yeah, it does worry me quite a bit,' I tell her. 'Especially with some stories in the media about women with my type of cancer having recurrences far into the future. It makes me wonder how long I'm going to be worrying about it and if I'll ever feel like I can relax. I read that recurrences for hormone positive breast cancer can happen really far down the track, so that was worrying.'

'Well, it's still most likely to happen within five years,' she tells me. 'But you're right, it does have a longer tail than most cancers. Do you want to see a psychologist?'

I say that I do, but I find the conversation quite abrupt and not in line with my expectations. Perhaps it is the fact that the clinic is running extremely late and my appointment starts fifty minutes later than the scheduled time, but I feel I am being rushed out of this conversation. Before I can ask about the research and request more information about my recurrence risk, I have been handed a referral for the psychology service at the hospital and gently nudged out the door.

The research highlights the importance of these oncologist-led interventions, which involve the offer to provide resources that give patients their individual risk profiles and outline symptoms to watch out for, ensuring people aren't worrying unnecessarily about every niggle in their body. It also calls for oncologists to talk through tactics for managing worry and provide links to online resources. Referral to a psychologist is recommended as the final step for patients whose fear is severe and are not able to be reassured by the other steps. I feel like I am being skipped straight to the end, which only heightens my worry. Does that mean my risk profile is so high that the oncologist does not want to offer to provide me that information? Am I coming across as highly fearful and in need of special psychological intervention? Later, when I am able to take the time to reflect on the appointment, I can see I was probably being a little unfair in my expectations. Every time I walk into the specialist cancer hospital – where all my treatment took place and where I still attend appointments – I can feel the stress levels in my body rise. That day I had also needed to visit the hospital pharmacy, which is housed just outside the day therapy ward, where chemo is administered. The sights and smells of the place had me on edge, so I probably had a heightened emotional response to my appointment not playing out in the exact way I had envisaged.

And so I try to put my worries aside and just go to see the psychologist. It helps a little, but I don't feel like my psychologist – even being a specialist onco-psychologist – is able to give me some of that targeted information. While she does help me get myself out of my own head and process the emotions of listening to other people's traumatic experiences, I don't find the sessions help manage my fear of recurrence. I can acknowledge the fear and come up with strategies to work through it, but I don't have the underlying statistical information that will help me rationalise through my worries. Maybe that's not something that everyone needs, but that rationalisation is a huge part of the way I weed out anxiety, so I feel a bit empty.

While I am unable to find the answers I need from health care professionals, I still have a desire to better understand the space this fear occupies and how to control it. I decide I need to hear the perspective of someone who lives with their deepest fears and has found a way to persist in the face of ongoing trauma.

Greg

I first met Greg Harris over thirty years ago, when I was the smallest kid in the kindergarten class at my primary school and he was the biggest teacher in the school. Standing at well over six feet tall, he seemed like a literal giant to my five-year-old self. He taught Year 6 and was known among the younger students to be 'scary'. For some reason, there was a fundraiser at the school that involved bringing labels in from Heinz cans – the more labels the school could collect, the more equipment they would receive from Heinz as a prize. So every week, my mum sent me off to school with a bunch of labels and I would need to take them to the teacher who was coordinating the school's entry – Mr Harris. The first few times I had to walk into his classroom, I was terrified. I begged my mum to forget about the Heinz labels, but that was never going to happen. My family has a deep competitive streak and competitions like this are irresistible to my mum and her siblings. So I faced my fears and walked into that classroom and handed them over. Each week, it got easier. Soon I realised that Mr Harris wasn't actually scary at all. He was always kind, welcoming and grateful that my family was taking the time to support the school.

A few years later, I decided to try out for the school cross-country team. Mr Harris was the sports coordinator and really encouraged me to keep on persisting, even though I wasn't the most athletic kid. He fostered within me a love of running and a desire for improvement, a lifelong gift. Mr Harris stopped teaching at our school when I was in my final years there, but his daughter was friends with my sister and over the years, he and his wife became close friends with my parents. He coached my sister's cricket team and our families spent a lot of time together – he and my parents are still close to this day. He became a family friend and I stopped thinking of him as Mr Harris and he simply became Greg.

A few days after my cancer diagnosis, my dad met up with Greg for lunch. By this stage, Greg had been dealing with his own cancer for a number of years, so he was immediately understanding. He listened to my dad's worries, gave advice when needed and provided great empathy in his typically kind and caring way. As I posted about my progress on social media, Greg kept in contact. Through his messages and comments, I always felt that he was there as a support person, as someone who understood what it was like to go through this. His cancer was much more difficult to treat than mine and he was dealing with his own extremely tough times. It would have been completely reasonable if he chose to switch off from my story, to feel it was unfair that I had this diagnosis of a cancer that could be easily treated and wasn't necessarily a death sentence. But he didn't. The message I received from Greg shortly after my diagnosis is one that stayed with me throughout the entire treatment process. It was rare to get the chance to speak to someone who understood, and who I didn't feel like I needed to protect from the realities of my fear and worry about what lay ahead.

> I can and can't imagine all that must be going through your thoughts at this time. It is indeed a physical and mental rollercoaster, but as the reality of it all begins to be

> understood bit by bit, I hope you reach an understanding and acceptance that this is what life has dealt you and you just have to get on with it. I appreciate you won't be here yet, but I hope the journey gets easier the more you understand. My own, very different journey with this and a family member also (who by the way has just come out with a clean bill of health) with everything you are about to begin does give me some perspective on your journey. We are thinking of you.

This simple message of acceptance, hope and resilience was exactly what I needed to hear at the time. It has shaped my own responses when people have confided about their illness or traumatic experiences in the time since. It taught me that what people need most in those moments is not advice or unfailing positivity but understanding.

I speak to Greg on the phone about a year after finishing my treatment. I want to thank him for his kindness and let him know about the impact it had on me. I also want to understand more about what he has been through.

Greg's journey began in November 2017, when he was coaching his school's basketball team on a Saturday morning. 'A little boy who was playing in the game got injured, and I ran out on the court and realised he needed to come off,' Greg says. 'So I went to pick him up and

I hurt my lower back. I was in excruciating pain, but I stayed for that game and the next game, and I went to my nephew's wedding in pain, and had a terrible night.'

When he went to the doctor, he discovered that he'd done some damage to his back and started the difficult process of making a workers' compensation claim to get the treatment he needed. However, his doctor of twenty years was reluctant to work with the insurance agencies and Greg needed to find a new general practitioner. As soon as the new doctor saw Greg's scans, she realised something more was going on. After multiple series of tests – during which time he discovered that he had eleven crush fractures in his vertebrae and had lost seven centimetres of height – he received a call from the doctor.

'The day she called me was actually a workday and she sent me for an ultrasound before work,' he says. 'They wanted to check if there were any infections going on in soft tissue. And on the way back from that ultrasound, I was heading to work and the doctor's receptionist rang and said, "The doctor wants you to pop in."'

It was then Greg found out that he had a rare blood cancer called multiple myeloma. After a quick explainer from the doctor, he headed into work, his head spinning from his world being turned upside down. 'It was the last week of school and that weekend, I was taking a group of boys to a big rugby tournament in Armidale,' he says. 'They knew I had been in terrible pain with my back for a long while and there was already some discussion about whether I should go.'

Greg spoke to his boss and the school counsellor about his diagnosis and was told that he had to make an announcement to the staff about what was going on. 'Up to that point, I think I'd been pretty good,' he says. 'But then they made me stand in front of the staff and tell them what I'd been told that morning. I lasted about a minute, and then I burst into tears and stormed out of the room. I just couldn't face them.'

Cancer began to consume Greg's life. Treatment has been a long and arduous process, as myeloma does not currently have a cure. But the hardest thing for him to face has been the impact on his family. His wife, daughter, son and two daughters-in-law are his world and experiencing their reactions has been devastating for him. 'We weren't sure how long I was going to be around for, what I'd get to experience, how many Christmases and birthdays that'd still be left for me,' he says. 'It was tough for everyone. My daughter worries an awful lot. She contacts me every couple of days to see how I'm going. My son locks his emotions away, but I know he worries about me too and I see the tears in his eyes at times.'

In all the time I have known Greg, it has always been incredibly clear to me how devoted he is to his family. The love he has for them runs deep and it seems to radiate out of his pores when he is with them. From coaching his daughter's and son's cricket teams with so much care and effort, to staying at parties much later than he would have liked because his wife was in her element, I've witnessed the way he continually puts them first in big and small ways. It is through this lens that I have always viewed Greg's connection to his family. He loves them deeply and takes his responsibility to them seriously. Listening to him talk about the way his illness has affected his family while he struggles to hold back tears is difficult and I wish I had the words to reassure him.

Greg had been undergoing treatment for two years when the Covid pandemic hit and the tightrope he was walking to try to keep his health in check suddenly got narrower and higher. Despite all the complications the pandemic caused for him – multiple instances of contracting Covid that compromised his care and delays to surgeries and other treatments – it was the physical separation from his family that caused the most distress. 'It was a nightmare,' he says. 'It was just a sense of loneliness, a sense of being dispossessed of your family. It was tough to not have that support at that time, although we obviously kept in contact with lots of text messaging and chatting.'

The birth of his first granddaughter in April 2021 was a time of love and celebration, but Sydney went back into lockdown when she was only three months old and suddenly, the few kilometres between them stretched out like an ocean. 'She was a blessing and she just brought so much joy, but suddenly to have these periods where we couldn't see her was tough,' he says. 'And even after lockdown ended, any time she got a cold or anyone was sick, they couldn't come near me. So it was very, very stressful.'

Greg's long stretch of pain and difficulty is ongoing. When we speak, he is frank about the fact that he is running out of options for treatment. Since his diagnosis, he has had multiple drugs, surgeries and other kinds of treatment to try to contain the myeloma. Each has worked for a period of time and then failed. His most successful treatment was part of a clinical trial, but contracting Covid and having some issues with his liver function results due to a gall bladder infection meant he had to come off it, and once he had been removed from the trial, he was not able to get back in.

'So what's happened now is there's not much left out there for me that my haematologist feels is going to be successful,' he says. 'He wanted to get me on to these CAR T-cell trials. CAR T is being hailed as possibly the cure for multiple myeloma at some point down the track, but it's still early stages. But just at the time that he wanted to get me into a trial, all the trials across Australia closed because they've reached maximum numbers. And that was maybe going to be the golden bullet for me.'

Our long discussion is incredibly emotional and while we talk, Greg's tears flow more than once. But while he tells me about his new treatment – a bispecific antibodies trial – he is hopeful and spirited. He is not finished fighting this beast and while he walks into every treatment with open eyes, knowing it may not work, he also keeps an open heart, hoping that it will. 'My first check-up for this latest treatment was a couple of days ago and I felt like nothing happened in that time, my tumours felt exactly the same, with the same amount of pain,' he says. 'But here I am, two days later. I spoke with a nurse today and there are actually some signs of some things improving. So fingers crossed, this may be the start of something happening with this treatment.'

Unlike me, Greg does not have the luxury of putting cancer – or the trauma he has been through – behind him. It is an inextricable part of him and has thrown his life into permanent disarray. 'As I get further down the track, I now fully accept that this cancer is going to kill me, I just don't know when,' he says matter-of-factly. 'I think I've worked through those Kubler-Ross stages of death – blaming, accepting and all that sort of stuff. We all have a use-by date. We don't spend a lot of time thinking about it, but suddenly when you have cancer, that use-by date is there in front of you like a flashing neon sign except unfortunately, you just can't see the final date on it.'

Despite the deep sadness at the heart of Greg's story, it is ultimately one about having the strength to build a life that is incredibly fulfilling and joyful in the toughest of circumstances. In the years since his diagnosis, his world has shrunk from being an active and busy teacher, impacting the lives of students through their academic and sporting pursuits, to narrowing his role down to being a husband, a father, a grandfather and a friend. While his sphere of influence is now much smaller, Greg still radiates that same love and energy out into the world and makes sure he directs it wherever it can be most helpful. 'I want to make sure I leave a positive legacy,' he says. 'My goal in life has always been to make sure wherever I have been, whenever I walk away, I've left it in a better state than it was when I started. I feel I've fulfilled that to the best of my ability, in everything from my family to the jobs that

I've done. I think I've reached out and given of myself way beyond my comfort zone.'

He tells me a story about his final day at school before retirement. He was working at a private boys' school, where he taught in the junior school. There were three teachers who were leaving after more than twenty years of service at the school, so Greg was expecting they would all be similarly honoured. 'When the principal just called me up to shake my hand and I turned around, the whole school was on their feet, all the high school boys who knew me, clapping and giving me a standing ovation. I was quite embarrassed.'

While the other two teachers received enthusiastic applause, they did not receive the same reaction as Greg, which surprised him. 'I didn't realise that I had made that sort of an impact,' he says. 'I really didn't appreciate it at the time. So I think my level of appreciation of moments like that has certainly risen.'

That night, Greg had a small farewell dinner with the other junior school teachers, during which his boss made a speech thanking Greg for his years of service and describing what made him such a special teacher. 'I was listening to two boys talking after assembly this afternoon – one of them had been through the junior school and one of them hadn't,' the principal told the group. 'The boy who hadn't been with us for junior school wanted to know why everyone rose to clap that teacher who was leaving. The other boy turned to him and said, "Oh, that's Mr Harris. He's a class act."'

Recalling this moment almost two years later, Greg is still rendered almost speechless with emotion. 'I didn't even know who the kid was, he didn't give me a name or anything,' he says. 'That's pretty special, that a kid would make that sort of a judgement about me. I've gone through my life wondering whether I really was making an impact, but now that I've got to this point, I think maybe I have made an impact on people and maybe the goodness that my parents instilled in me has shone through. My mother always said to look for the good in people and I've followed that advice right through my life.'

For the past few months before our chat, Greg's focus had been on attending his daughter's wedding. However, he was coming off an extremely difficult twelve months of treatments working for a short while and then failing. It appeared the myeloma was beginning to win the battle over his body and treatment options were becoming harder to find. His haematologist was painting a less-than-promising diagnosis for the future.

'He had started telling me that things were getting very serious,' Greg says. 'The cancer had moved out of my blood and bones and had begun to appear in the soft tissue of my body. I had about six painful plasmacytomas throughout my body and more hidden internally along my spine.' Greg had been undergoing radiation to try to get the plasmacytomas – tumours made up of abnormal plasma cells – under control, but it didn't work. Eventually, the sheer number of tumours meant radiation became unrealistic.

'I really started to feel like the cancer was completely taking hold of my body,' he says. 'My haematologist recommended a heavy-duty chemotherapy treatment where I'd go into hospital and get multiple chemotherapy drugs at once to try and get the cancer back under control. He was hoping this would give him time to find a new treatment or trial drug that could be more successful. It was looking quite grim.'

This treatment was extremely aggressive and toxic and was more than likely going to make Greg very sick and even threaten his life. It ended up doing both, keeping him in hospital for over a month as infectious disease doctors, surgeons and haematologists fought to control an infection caused by the treatment and cancer all at once.

Throughout this time, Greg remained determined that he would make it to the wedding, even as he got sicker and the infections got worse. The doctors and nurses assured

Greg they were working their hardest to get him to the wedding, but they weren't able to make any promises.

Through the dedication and determination of Greg's medical team – as well as sheer willpower on his part – both the infection and cancer were brought under control enough to permit him to leave hospital for the day to make the one-hour trip down to Wollongong – just south of Sydney – to see his daughter and her new wife celebrate their love.

'They'd been engaged for four years and it was taking so long that we never thought it was going to happen,' he says, smiling. 'So to then have it lined up with this time where they had to throw me into hospital to try and control this cancer, I was worried that I wouldn't make it down there. But in the end, they got me to that wedding, they let me go out in the morning,' he says. 'I got all dressed up and they stuck me in a wheelchair. We had the most beautiful day and before the day ended, I was back in the hospital bed again. It was surreal.'

The difficulties he had faced in the lead-up to the wedding slipped completely off his shoulders when he arrived and the excitement and joy of the celebration took over. 'I was just so glad to be there, so proud of my daughter. I said to her, "Am I going to walk you down the aisle?" It was in a little courthouse and the aisle wasn't very long. She said,

"Oh, I forgot all about that, Dad, do you want to walk me down the aisle?"'

Although Greg had not been on his feet in weeks, his leg scarred with damage and pain, he was determined that he wanted to share this walk with his daughter. 'She held on to me and I walked her down the twenty-metre aisle of this old courthouse and I gave her a kiss and off they went and got married,' he says. 'It was one of the proudest days of my life to be able to do that for her.'

While so much is now out of his control, Greg continues to hold on to these moments of bliss with his family.

At the centre of it all is his wife, with whom he spends every day. 'My great joy every day is to wake up and see her,' he says. 'I thought I loved her when I first met her, but I love her even more now. I love to see her every day. I love to spend time with her. Some days we have very quiet days. We don't say a lot, but just to know she's nearby is enough. I try not to ask much of her. She was always offering, but I learned to say no, because I don't want her to do too much for me. I just want to spend time with her. She is the most incredible human being – quiet, gentle, but so, so strong.'

Despite being in a holding pattern as he waits to see if his latest treatment will be effective and what quality of life it may offer him, Greg is generally a positive and resolute person. His words to me following my diagnosis come trickling back – this is truly what it means to face trauma with 'understanding and acceptance'.

When we speak about his outlook on life, Greg is thoughtful. He has plenty of time on his hands these days and he has pieced together an approach to living with cancer that allows him to focus on the joys in his life without ever really forgetting that he is deeply embedded in trauma. 'Through my years of teaching and coaching, I can focus and compartmentalise things, I can push problems away and put them in a little corner of my mind and just live for the things that I love,' he says. 'I find joy in every day. I enjoy my wife's company, we laugh every day, we chat every day. I get to talk to my kids. I love the sun shining through my window or sitting out on the front porch, walking around our beautiful garden, doing little things where I can. On the days where I've got the energy to do some work around the house, I really enjoy being able to contribute.'

The sadness sits just below the surface and while he doesn't bottle it up, he also doesn't let it overwhelm him. Some days, that is easier than others. Something as simple as a story on the news can cause the tears to spill over, but these moments can also be cathartic. 'I guess the question is, what is strength?' he asks. 'Strength is accepting the challenges you've got and then getting on with life and making the most of things. I don't want to be a sad sack that just sits around at home and says, "Woe is me". I've never been that sort of person.'

When it comes to confronting his challenges, Greg feels that he is constantly drawing on life experience that has made him the person he is. 'I remember watching my kids play cricket and they'd get hit by that junior cricket ball which is basically a plastic ball and they'd cry. And then they move up the grades and they end up playing with the hard ball and they'd get hit and come home with a bruise on their leg the size of a grapefruit. But when you watched them get hit, they didn't flinch. You learn how to manage pain in your life through painful events. I think all the things I've been through, from the death of parents and family members, through to my own personal injuries from sport and other things, I think we learn how to manage pain and shelve it away and compartmentalise it in ways which I find very hard to understand at times.'

Most of all, Greg just wants to live. He wants to be there to see his granddaughter grow up, to talk to his children and laugh with his wife. 'I often think about people who consider suicide. I know they've got a whole lot of mental health issues going on,' he says. 'But I think, here I am at sixty-two. I just want to live longer and people are making decisions to take their lives. I can never understand that. I want to be here for as long as I can, to enjoy my life and enjoy my family and whatever each day has to offer me. I can never quite understand people whose life has got so bad that they feel the need to check out at such a young age. I find that so sad.'

When I speak to Greg about the kindness he showed me during my diagnosis and treatment, it's another emotional moment. I ask him what motivated him to reach out amid his own difficult time and he does not hesitate. 'I just felt like I just needed to say something to support you,' he says. 'I could feel your pain, I can empathise with what you're going through and the uncertainty of it. You've got a beautiful daughter, a husband, your beautiful life and you're watching it slip away. I just wanted to reach out to say hang in there. It's amazing what they can do. And, for you, the story so far looks like it's been a very positive one. But it wasn't necessarily going to be that way, it's not necessarily going to be that way for me. But every time you help others, you grow a little bit yourself. So there's a method to the madness.'

Greg's story is difficult to hear. While everyone I speak to carries their trauma with them to a certain extent, for Greg, there is no moving on. There is no moment in time that he can forget about what has happened to him.

Cancer is likely a part of his life forever, and he will be continually working to kick it a little further down the road. While I will carry my fear of recurrence and the 'scanxiety' that accompanies me at my annual ultrasound and mammogram for the rest of my life, Greg's burden is much heavier.

From the moment I was diagnosed, people have told me I am brave, inspirational and strong. When someone dies from cancer, the obituaries are full of proclamations that they have 'lost their battle'. This language has always felt wrong to me and my friend Josephine Tovey – who had bowel cancer at the same time I had breast cancer – sums up so neatly why it doesn't sit well with cancer patients: 'Cancer patients get a lot of praise for bravery but it's not like you have a choice,' she writes. 'Far from a battle you arm up for, I found cancer to be a disease that renders you passive, immediately – something to accept and yield to.'[24]

Having listened to Greg's story, what strikes me as key to the way he has shaped his life in the painful years since his diagnosis is the acceptance. It is contained in the message he sent me, and it has been threaded quietly through the way he lives his life.

I go back to his words again: 'I hope you reach an understanding and acceptance that this is what life has dealt you and you just have to get on with it.'

To those who have not been through it, these words may seem harsh and lacking in empathy. But to me, they immediately resonated. Everything had happened so quickly and I was deep in survival mode. I didn't feel brave or strong, and when people sent encouragement in the form of 'you got this', I felt immediately disconnected, because I was certain that I absolutely did not have this. But something I felt I could manage was to accept what had happened and get on with it. I could put my head down and go to appointments on my own because the pandemic precluded me from bringing a support person. I could get through having my body cut open, injected with poison and beamed with radiation. There was nothing I could do to fight or be active in this process. But acceptance and getting on with it? That I could do.

The other thing that stays with me from my discussion with Greg is the idea of compartmentalising. My own lack of emotional reaction to my diagnosis and all that I have been through since has continued to trouble me, but the way Greg speaks about his ability to 'push problems away and put them in a little corner of (his) mind' as a positive way to manage his emotional state has given me something to think about. Maybe the worries, fears and big emotions that lie hidden in the locked boxes of my own mind are okay to stay there for a while. Perhaps they won't necessarily explode open one day and overwhelm me, but, like Greg, I may just be able to open them a crack from time to time and set some of those emotions free. It makes me realise that the fear I have of being overwhelmed by emotion, and experiencing a complete breakdown, has led to me suppress my emotions even further.

The numbness that I felt throughout my treatment has started to eke away and there have been times when I start to feel those emotions trickling through. But I keep pushing them back, afraid that they will lead to a tidal wave I cannot control. I believed it must be all or nothing. Greg has taught me that I can feel sadness, fear and worry – not just experience it intellectually, but actually *feel* it – without succumbing to it. I can let the tears come when I feel sad, exhausted or proud without it necessarily meaning that I will be wiped out for days in an emotional turmoil.

And even if the breakdown does happen, I will manage it. After all, I have managed so much else.

CHAPTER THREE

Bury Me Deep in Love

'Life gives us our toughest challenges when we need them.'

I realise at one point that I am basing my idea of what a healthy emotional response is on my nine-year-old daughter. Ever since she was tiny, her teachers have told us, 'Pia has big emotions.' And it's true: Pia feels things deeply. To a lot of people, that can just look like tears at what they deem to be inappropriate times, or 'overreacting' to situations. But Pia's emotions occupy the full range of the spectrum – when she's happy or excited, she lights up a room and fills whatever space she's in with joy. Unfortunately, that side is not often acknowledged.

She's told she needs to be more 'resilient' because people feel uncomfortable letting her sit with her negative emotions.

It is something I have noticed a lot since becoming a parent, that we as a society do not like to see children expressing negative emotions. I have witnessed many responses to my daughter's tears, from distraction to ordering her to 'stop crying' and none of them have been remotely useful or effective. I suspect the reason for this discomfort stems from the same place as responses we have to other people's trauma. People are frightened of emotion and don't know how to deal with it when it comes at them in floods. As adults, we have learnt to conceal our big, negative emotions and we expect children to do the same. Allowing Pia to feel her feelings, however, has always been a conscious choice for Shaun and me. The truth is that she is incredibly resilient, much more than I am. When she experiences something that upsets her, she works through it by letting those emotions happen, which often involves crying. But once she has done that, she can move on. It doesn't mean that she no longer has any sadness about the situation, but she's also able to let other feelings in, like happiness for a friend or looking forward to something else in the future.

I figure out that what I wish I had done during my experience with cancer was to process my emotions like she does. Although it wouldn't earn me the same kind of praise I'd got for the way I did react – people telling me I was 'strong' or 'brave' or 'positive' – I need to reframe my own idea of resilience away from those expectations. I need the emotional health of a nine-year-old.

Pia was seven when I was diagnosed and she was the second person I told, after Shaun. How and when I told her about it is always one of the first questions I am asked. Some people tell me that they would have hidden it from their kids, had it happened to them. For me, that was never an option. Pia is at the centre of my life. You only have to spend a few minutes in my presence to know that I am absolutely obsessed with this child. I spend more time with her than anyone else in the world. When I was going through treatment, Shaun worked weekends, so Pia and I were a little unit on Saturdays and Sundays, always together. There was no way I was going to have this hugely significant thing hit my life and not share it with her. Shaun and I were completely on the same page. He sat near me while I spoke to my GP on the phone in the backyard and heard the news that was about to change my life forever. We spent about ten minutes talking it over and immediately headed inside to tell Pia.

'Can we talk to you for a second?' I asked her. She looked up from her drawing warily. 'You know how I've been having some tests and doctors' appointments to figure out what this lump in my breast is?'

'Yes,' she said. 'Do you know what it is now?'

'Yes,' I told her. 'Unfortunately, the lump is breast cancer. Have you heard of cancer before?'

'I think so,' she said. 'Is it something really bad?'

'It's a pretty serious illness,' I said. 'You might hear stories about people who die from cancer. But the kind of cancer I have is one that they have lots of treatments for. I have really good doctors and they're going to work really hard and get this all fixed. The treatment can be pretty rough, but it's worth it. I'll get through all this and we'll be able to go on with our lives.'

We chatted some more; I gave all the reassurances I could and tried not to bombard her with information. Pia was old enough to understand what was happening, but young enough that she didn't question the idea that I was going to be okay. She had complete trust in Shaun and me and believed us when we said that I would get through this.

The question I still get asked the most is how Pia has coped with it all. I did have concerns that she may react badly at some point. I made sure her teachers were aware of what was happening in case anything came out at school. But that trust and healthy processing of emotions haven't really shifted. There have certainly been disappointments – probably the most acute one when we weren't able to go to the Easter Show in 2022 – but each time something came up, she cried her tears and felt her feelings and we were able to get past it. She sat reading in pathology waiting rooms while I had weekly blood tests and she came to my final chemo session, where she helped me ring the bell that indicated I had finished that portion of my treatment.

Pia became so intrinsically tangled in my experience that I found it hard to understand the effect that being a parent had on my trauma and in turn the effect trauma has had on my parenting. There were many parts of life I was simply not able to opt out of because my child needed me. In some ways, it helped me to continue, but it may have also pushed me further into survival mode, holding me back from processing my trauma fully.

I am certainly not alone in feeling this way. For those who experience trauma before becoming parents, this can be a huge factor in their decision to have – or not have – children. Gina Rushton explores the complexities associated with this decision in her book, *The Most Important Job in the World*. Through her interviews with a number of different people who sit on all sides of the fence on this issue, she illustrates the worries, struggles and joy of the interweaving of trauma and parenting.

> I want to believe that the hardest moments in life tilt like a series of dominoes falling from one generation into the next, and if we try hard enough we can catch the falling tile

> before it hits another. I want to believe this even though I know the precursor cell of the egg I developed from was already in my mother's ovaries when she was a five-month-old foetus, curled up in my grandmother's womb.[25]

Rushton also considers the ramifications of epigenetics – the study of how external factors like behaviour and environment can change the way the body reads a DNA sequence and make physiological changes to people.

'Epigenetics is where nurture and nature meet to offer a different flavour of fatalism on the journey to answer the question of how much I will fuck up any potential offspring,' she writes. 'It suggests you can pass on your genes and then adversely impact how those genes are expressed.'

The Center on the Developing Child at Harvard University explains that while epigenetics is still an emerging field of study, most research supports the idea that children's brains are the most susceptible to epigenetic changes.

'Injurious experiences, such as malnutrition, exposure to chemical toxins or drugs, and toxic stress before birth or in early childhood are not "forgotten", but rather are built into the architecture of the developing brain through the epigenome,' the Center reports. 'The "biological memories" associated with these epigenetic changes can affect multiple organ systems and increase the risk not only for poor physical and mental health outcomes but also for impairments in future learning capacity and behaviour.'[26]

Essentially, when a traumatic experience occurs in childhood, it manifests in the body of the child as a kind of physical memory and remains there as they age. These bodily memories of trauma can increase the likelihood that a person will experience physical and mental illnesses and learning difficulties.

While this realisation seems scary at first, it also feels almost empowering somehow. The more we learn about epigenetic changes, the more support can be offered to parents and children to help counteract these deep impacts of trauma. The Center on the Developing Child notes that recent research suggests that it may be possible to reverse some negative changes to the way DNA is read, but even without this advancement, simply having the knowledge of epigenetic changes taking place will allow greater understanding and support for those impacted by intergenerational trauma.

This knowledge has helped me to come to terms with some of the ways in which trauma intersects with my parenting and effects that are both inside and outside of my control. But I feel the pull to discuss this more deeply with someone who has experience of parenting after trauma.

Emily

I've known Emily for almost ten years and we clicked immediately. On the surface, we are very different people – she is ten years younger than me and grew up in the country, where she dealt with severe childhood trauma. But despite our differences, our bond grew, and when our daughters were born close together and we found ourselves in the new motherhood trenches, we built a genuine friendship. Emlly is kind, funny, opinionated and empathetic – all qualities I value deeply. These days, she lives back up in the country with her husband and their two daughters, so we don't see each other often. But those early years of navigating new motherhood together created a bond between us that will always be there.

We speak late at night, both of us tired from the day and getting our daughters to bed. Emily's second child is still just a toddler. I remember the more arduous process of getting smaller children into bed and I don't envy her that. We talk on the phone, over 300 kilometres apart, haltingly at first as we rediscover our rhythms, then falling back into our old patterns.

Emily's childhood was defined by violence. She describes running down to the back paddock with her younger brother to hide when her father became violent at home. She had trouble forming friendships at school because she felt insecure about her old shoes and clothes that smelled of cigarette smoke. She found it hard to concentrate because there was never enough to eat at home. She has no childhood memories from before she was eight years old. She describes the state she was in as a kind of dissociation. 'It was almost like putting on a front, pretending that life was great and nothing was going on,' she says. 'The night before we'd have gone through absolute hell and back, and I'd still have to get up, get myself ready for school, go spend a solid day at school with everyone and then get on the bus and then go home.'

Emily felt like she had an internal switch that she would flick on when she got on the bus each morning, becoming the person she wanted to be at school, the person she felt like she had to be to get through the day. Each afternoon, when she stepped off the bus, the switch would turn back off. 'When I hopped off the bus it was like, here we go, back to reality,' she says. 'At school, I felt like I had to fit in and be this other person and it wasn't someone I could be when I got off the bus. I wasn't happy. I was hypervigilant all the time, just thinking about what could happen next, what would that night be like?'

Emily's oldest sister moved in with their grandparents when Emily was eight and the three children left at home did their best to stay out of harm's way. 'My other sister usually hid when things were happening, so I would have to take my little brother, and we ran down to the back paddock,' she says. 'I always felt like I had to protect him because he would want to protect Mum. But then I also had to make sure that my sister was okay.'

Over the years, the situation at home progressively became worse and Emily and her siblings started to run away further – often to the diner a few kilometres from their home, where they could use the payphone to call their grandmother. Other times their grandmother would arrive on their doorstep to take them away for the night, particularly if the police had been called. 'Nan would come and get us and we'd go away for the night and then we'd come back the next day,' she says. 'So we'd get away for a bit but then we'd always have to return. It wasn't until I was almost fifteen, when I was at school one day and Department of Community Services (DOCS) came in and asked to have a meeting and an interview with me and my brother. Then gradually over the course of the year, things started to move and progress toward living at Nan's.'

Even once she had moved, it took some time before Emily felt safe in her new home. The hypervigilance she had experienced over many years had taken a toll on her mind and body. 'I think it took me a while because, even though they'd said we were going to our grandparents' place and we didn't have to go home, it still very much felt like I was going to get picked up one day and taken home,' she says. 'It was always in the back of my mind that they'd made a mistake, and they were going to undo it.'

It wasn't a feeling that left her until she was nineteen, even though she had moved away from home to start university a year before. The feelings of fear and impermanence were so ingrained that they took quite a lot of work to unlearn. It was a combination of self-reflection, supportive friends and family and psychological support that helped her overcome her doubts and feel comfortable. The psychological support was a difficult step. 'My nan doesn't believe in counselling or therapy, so when we first came into her care, I didn't get it.' she says. 'But when I moved to Sydney I had these really intense emotions and I thought to myself, "You know what? I'm actually going to give it a go, I'm gonna go to therapy, and I'm gonna sit down with someone and really talk about things."'

Emily's psychologist used a type of cognitive therapy that incorporated a metronomic beat to help address the symptoms and causes of the PTSD she was suffering. 'Every time the metronome would tick, I had to bring up what I was thinking at the time.' she says. 'So she'd start with a topic and then I'd have to bounce off that. A lot of the time it would dive into that PTSD and talking through what happened to me as a kid. I got so much out of that.'

Despite all that she went through, she has created a life for her two children that could not be further from what she experienced. 'I now look at my own family and I just think, "Oh my god, this is reality",' she tells me. 'This is what a magazine page of a family looks like, two kids, a husband, a house, all that stuff.'

It has been a long and often difficult path for her to reach this point. She felt a lot of fear and anxiety around parenting, felt that she had to make conscious choices to build a childhood very different from the one she experienced. This was compounded by the fact that her pregnancy came unexpectedly, when she was only twenty years old and not yet finished university. 'When I was pregnant, I would often get upset that I wasn't doing enough for [her eldest child],' she says. 'I wanted to do the conventional stuff, because that was drilled into me by my nan – you get married, you buy a house, you have a good job, and then you have kids. So it was kinda like, "Shit, this isn't the life that I imagined."'

Despite the difficulties, Emily and her partner were determined to make it work. 'I knew I wasn't ready,' she says. 'But life gives us our toughest challenges when we need them. I reflect back and I would get quite upset, thinking to myself, I'm not going to be a good mum, I'm going to turn out to be like my parents. I can't do this. I can't provide for her and I can't do the things that I should be able to do for her. I don't know how to be a parent. All those emotions were very much there for at least the first four years of her life.'

It was a hard road, but she has got to the point where she feels like she can support others through the same journey. Her younger brother leaned on her for support when his wife was pregnant and he felt the doubts start to creep in. 'When they were going through pregnancy he would talk to me a lot about our childhood,' Emily says. 'He often asked me, how did I parent, how did I get over the feelings that we had when we were kids.'

Like Emily, her brother worried that the trauma he had faced in his childhood would impact his own children. He wasn't sure he knew how to be a parent in the way that he wanted to be. 'He was really worried that he was gonna turn out to be a father like our father,' Emily says. 'He had a lot of anger and sadness about that. So I would have weekly phone calls with him around that time. I was almost like his counsellor at that point.'

The most important lesson Emily could impart was one of self-acceptance and love. 'Something that kids do to us is they make us see who we really are,' she says. 'Me and my brother, we're not the monsters that we thought we would have been with what happened to us. He's doing amazing as a parent – I knew he would, but he didn't always know. I think he believes it now though.'

Emily has kept in touch with therapy at key points in her life – her move back to her hometown sparked a recurrence in feelings of fear, as she worried about her parents trying to become involved in her life now that she was living close by. 'I felt very hypervigilant 24/7,' she says. 'It was even like, what if I run into the people that they used to hang out with – things like that. So I found a psychologist nearby and went through that for a year, which helped me process all those feelings.'

In late 2022, Emily again reached out for support through Victims Services, when turmoil around her youngest brothers – who are still living at home with her parents – started to swirl around her. 'I didn't realise that counselling for victims of crime was a thing, nobody had told me about it,' she says. 'I applied for it and got twenty counselling sessions. I've been doing that to give myself a chance to sit in this space now. A lot's happening and I've realised that my little brothers (born after Emily had left home) may eventually come to live with us and I'm going to have to deal with my parents again. They're going to be in my life, because that's part of having the kids, making sure that they have family time and contact.'

It is a stark reminder of the continual touchpoints a traumatic event has, the long, winding roots that spread out beneath a life where trauma has grown. Emily survived; she made it out of an awful situation and has built a life for herself that is far from what she experienced in her youth. She found a way – many ways in fact – to move on and put it all behind her. But it still finds a way to keep coming back. It is not something that can be conquered all at once, but requires patience and an acceptance of the inevitability of facing the problem again and again.

While Emily and I have been through different types of trauma, common themes emerge around the way it intersects with parenting. She has had the same kind of questions come up around how to talk to her children about what has happened to her. This has been a more gradual process than it was for me, because violence is not easy to explain. Her oldest daughter has started to ask more questions about Emily's parents and her relationship with them.

'When she was younger, when there'd be a big family gathering at Easter or Christmas, she used to ask, "Why don't they come and see me?"' Emily remembers. 'I had to explain to her, when mummy was little, they weren't very nice people. They did a lot of not very nice stuff to each other and to us. And that meant that we had to go live with Nan and Poppy when we were a bit older.'

I recognise this careful navigation around violence in Amani Haydar's powerful memoir *The Mother Wound*.[27] Haydar describes her own conversation with her daughter in the wake of her mother's death at the hands of her father: 'My daughter asks about my father. "Where's your baba?" "He lives far away," I answer. "Why don't you visit him?" "Because I am not friends with him anymore," I answer, carefully. "Sometimes big people do really bad things or make us really, really sad. When they do, it is okay to stop being friends with them."'

Explaining violence to children is not easy and, as such, this careful navigation feels essential – giving children enough information to understand why something is so, but in such a way as to not scare or worry them needlessly. It is something no parent knows how to do innately, but many unfortunately must figure out as they go.

As Emily's daughter has grown, she has begun to understand more about the tension and distance in her extended family and is starting to comprehend the enormity of it. 'She realises that what they've done in the past has hurt all of us quite a lot,' Emily says. 'And that it's something obviously big enough for us to not forgive them. So she recognises it, but I haven't actually gone into depth.

If she ever asks when she's much older, I could go into depth. But right now, she just knows that they did a lot of wrong stuff by us and they weren't very kind parents.'

While her trauma is not something that will ever leave her completely, Emily has reached a point in her life where it is no longer her defining feature. In her new life as a parent to two incredible daughters, she has redefined what a family means, as well as redefining herself in her new life. 'Coming from such a big family, one of eight kids, we didn't connect with anybody, we were just living,' she says, 'And I look at that and think to myself, that's not what a family is. We were just surviving and we were so dependent on each other as kids.'

In contrast, Emily now feels surrounded by family – not just her husband and daughters, but her grandparents, brothers, sisters and her large family of in-laws, from the parents-in-law who live nearby, her husband's sister, aunties, uncles and cousins who love them all too. It feels like a new beginning. 'Getting to have the family that matters around and who are actively involved in your life and the ones who your kids make memories with – it's just been so nice to realise that this is normal,' she says. 'And I don't have to be worried or scared anymore. '

Becoming a parent has also given Emily the perspective to reflect on her younger self and the kind of parent she needed back then. With her oldest child now eight years old – the age Emily's memories go back to – she thinks about what she would say to her eight-year-old self. 'I would tell her that it's going to be okay,' she says slowly, thinking deeply about it. 'It's going to be hard but it's going to be okay. I would tell her that she's gonna go far and she's gonna do big things even if she's scared and still has a bit of fear in her. I'd tell her to speak up even louder and tell her to find the people who were looking out for her and really speak up to them and make a big thing of it, tell them what was really happening and what was really going on.'

While that eight-year-old version of herself missed out on a childhood, Emily does not seem to hold much resentment. Her focus instead is on making sure her own children get the experiences that she missed out on and, more importantly, avoid the experiences that forced her to dissociate from the world around her. 'All I know is that I want them to do what they want to do, I don't ever want to make them feel like they have to do certain things, because I've said so,' she says. 'I don't ever want them to fear that Dad's gonna hurt Mum – and they never have, which is the best life ever.'

But there still remains the lingering doubt, one that most parents experience, but that becomes more heightened in the wake of trauma. 'Always in the back of my mind, and still to this day, I think I should be doing more with them,' she admits. 'We should be doing this, and we shouldn't be doing that, I should be giving them the world.'

Emily knows these worries will never truly dissipate for her, but the work she has done to process everything that has happened in her past helps her to keep them under control and to remember that she is giving her children exactly what they need. 'They're beautiful kids, as wild as they are, they're beautiful,' she says. 'They're the best kids ever. So I think I must be doing something right. But it's still something I feel every now and again, but I also know that it's never going to happen for them, because I'll never let it happen.'

I know in my heart that I will never stop worrying about the effects of my trauma on Pia. For while I honestly answer that she has dealt so well with it all to everyone who asks, I can't say for sure where those twisted stems will take root in her. What effect having a mother who couldn't raise herself from bed may have on her down the track, whether the unlimited screen time I allowed to get us both through those tough days will rear its head in some ugly form in the future. It seems like a silly thing to worry about, but nevertheless it plays on my mind almost constantly. It is a more intense version of the guilt that many mothers experience – about whether we are doing enough for our children, if we are feeding them well enough, loving them enough. The addition of trauma into this equation turns that 'mother guilt' up a notch and leaves me feeling ill at ease.

When the subject of Pia's resilience is raised now, I find myself feeling angry. I want to yell and scream, 'I don't care that she cried because she wasn't in a group with her friends for an activity! Do you know what she's been through?' But I don't, because that is not me. I smile, I sweep the conflict aside and I promise to work on her resilience.

I learn a lot from listening to Emily – although I have known her for a long time now, we had never delved into that trauma from her past before. I was aware of it on a surface level, but until I had gone through something huge myself, I didn't feel comfortable asking about it. I'm so glad I eventually did. Emily too found some peace in that conversation and has told me since that it made her think about her childhood slightly differently and see the ramifications of her trauma from new angles.

Through our conversation I now understand that even once I process my own trauma and get myself to that next stage of my life, it will never truly be over. That sounds scary, but I'm convinced that it's actually okay. Because I don't know if I want to go back to being the person I was before, the parent I was before. Rather than wipe the slate clean, I can embrace the changes in me and the way my recovery has forced me to reckon with my own emotional responses. It has helped me reframe the way Pia responds to emotional situations and it can make me better at advocating for her when people do not understand that her emotions are valid and appropriate.

Emily has also given me a lot to think about in the way conversations with children about trauma can evolve as they grow up. One of the biggest flaws in my parenting is sometimes treating Pia as an adult, a peer, a friend. I am eager to introduce her to new experiences, books or movies that I love and sometimes rush in before she is ready. Perhaps I have done this to some extent with what I have shared about my trauma. I know I have certainly intensified the introduction of new experiences and pop culture since my diagnosis. There is some part of me that is hurrying her into growing up because I now live in deep awareness of my own mortality, perhaps subconsciously believing that there are things I must experience with her now because I may not get the chance in the future. It is an understandable reaction, but one that I need to try to fight.

Emily's words highlighted the importance of letting children have a childhood whenever we can. During the depths of a traumatic experience, that is often not possible, but as I inch toward my way to go on in the world, I know that I can learn from this and become more thoughtful with my parenting as I grow.

CHAPTER FOUR

I Won't Let You Go

'Be a sparkling unicorn in a world of jackasses.'

What can I do to help?

If you have ever been unlucky enough to find yourself immersed in a traumatic experience, you will know that this is the one sentence that echoes through your life again and again. It's a completely natural response – humans want to help each other. Our first instinct is to seek out the ways in which someone needs help and try to fulfil them. I have uttered these words many times when friends and family members had been going through tough times. But it wasn't until they came at me like an unrelenting wave that I understood the trouble they can cause.

I have no doubt that even bringing this up will make it seem as if I am ungrateful, so let me be clear: I appreciated every single offer of help. The fact that people cared enough to want to do something for me was incredible. But I found the question overwhelming – I had no idea what I wanted or needed in that moment. And although it was no-one's intention, the constant nature of the question began to feel like a demand. Time and again it was thrown at me until I felt buried by it. As an incurable people-pleaser, I felt like I needed to give them something to do, but was simultaneously terrified that if it wasn't the 'right' thing they would be upset and offended.

In the time since my recovery, I have again found myself in situations where people I care about are in crisis. Every time it happens, I have to physically pull my hands back from getting out my phone to text *What can I do to help?*. It's an almost unstoppable urge. So I get it, I really do. But now I force myself to stop and think about the lessons I learned when I was the one on the receiving end of the barrage of requests.

One memory stands out more than most. I was at home alone recovering from my first surgery. My husband was at work and my daughter was being cared for by my parents. I was feeling a bit fragile – still shell-shocked from the diagnosis and the whirlwind of being swept into the system, cut open, sewn up and sent home. I was on the couch, watching *Gilmore Girls* – the television show equivalent of being wrapped in a warm blanket and hugged – when my phone buzzed with a text from a friend: *I've made you a meal that you can freeze for when you need it. I'll drop it around today – I can come in and hang out for a bit if you're up to it or I can just leave it by the door for you.*

It's hard for me to imagine a more perfect offer than that. My friend managed to remove all but the simplest choices, so that all I had to decide was whether I was up to having company or not. I didn't have to tell her what kind of help I needed. I didn't even have to tell her what food to make. She didn't make me feel as if I would be offending her if I turned down the offer of her company. As it turned out, I did feel like hanging out with someone and that afternoon helped me so much. Food is such a universally good and helpful thing that it's hard to go wrong. Friends who were close by dropped off home-cooked meals that could be easily frozen. Those who were further away sent vouchers for meal delivery services or hampers of treats. There is very little that can go wrong in life that food won't make slightly better.

When I look beyond food, I think about things that would have helped me if I had been capable of processing the information and asking for them. Lifts to appointments to avoid the nightmare of hospital parking. Hanging out with my daughter and giving her the emotional attention that I just could not muster. An offer to sit and watch trashy TV with me while talking about nothing in particular. Sharing some meaningless gossip. Sending me photos of pets. TV and podcast recommendations. Voice messages from people I missed.

These are the ideas I look at to help people going through trauma. There is not much I can do to take away the pain or difficulty. They are in the middle of a desert and my choices are to reach down and take away a few grains of sand or to bring some extra sand along and sprinkle it on top. Neither seem to make much difference in the moment, but if everyone chooses one or the other, together we either meaningfully ease their suffering or add to their burden.

Overall, I think the most important thing to do for someone who is going through something huge is be there for the long run. That first moment is when everyone rallies around you. It's the big, breaking news story and support comes from all directions. But trauma lingers long after the flowers stop arriving. There comes a point when you post an update on social media and can almost physically feel the sighs from people as they scroll past. Where once you gathered likes and heartwarming comments, the lack now seems to say, 'Are you *still* going on about that?'

And so you withdraw. You stop talking about it, only daring to bring it up if someone asks. You are yesterday's news and the news cycle stops for no-one. You are left to quietly pick up the pieces as best you can. Perhaps this is all in my head and people do continue to care, but there is a distinct lack of engagement that feels significant and is difficult to process after the cascades of love that come around the time of the traumatic event.

I wanted to understand how other people had navigated this period of trauma. It was one of my roadblocks to moving on – the fact that I didn't feel like I had the 'right' to talk about it anymore, that no-one would be interested. Soon after finishing my treatment, I conducted some online workshops for young people with cancer through the charity Canteen – helping them learn how to tell their story in the media. At the end of the final workshop, three of us were left and spent some time chatting. The two young people had both finished their treatment years earlier and I was struck by how much they wanted to talk about it. Simply having the time and space to tell their story to strangers who were genuinely interested became this beautifully healing moment. Sometimes the greatest thing someone can do is continue to care after everyone else stops.

The idea of friendship and what it means to truly be there for someone became central for me, and I decided to speak to someone who had navigated extremely tough times and found the love and support of friends to be a crucial part of recovery.

Heather

I talk to Heather Reid on the phone one evening after dinner. Our lives are worlds apart – she lives in the Sunshine Coast hinterland on a property with her partner, Pam. Calling from my tiny apartment in Sydney and listening to her describe her lush surrounds, it seems strange that we are even in the same country.

Heather and I have never met in real life, but we have connected on Twitter. The social media platform is often maligned for its toxicity, but I hold a soft spot for it because I have found so many of my people there. Heather is one of those people – a woman working in the tough, male-dominated environment of sport. Through Twitter, many of us have found each other and have carved out communities and friendships. Women with passions for different sports have intersected and taught each other about our own sports and learned about other people's. Friendships have blossomed and people have met up at women's sporting events across Australia and the world.

Heather's sport is football – the kind that sometimes goes by soccer in Australia. Her history in the sport is long and intertwined with the very fabric of women's football in this country. She was involved in the formation of the Australian National University Women's Soccer Club in 1978 and the Australian Capital Territory Women's Soccer Association in 1979. Heather was appointed manager of the national women's team in 1984 and joined the Australian Women's Soccer Association (AWSA) Board the same year. In 1986 she was appointed the National Executive Director of the AWSA, a position she held until 1993. In 2004 she became the CEO of Capital Football (the governing body of football in the Australian Capital Territory), which made her the first female CEO of a state football federation. It was a role she held until her retirement in 2016. During her time as CEO, she was instrumental in obtaining a licence for Canberra United to join the Australian professional women's competition. She was also part of the local organising committee for the 2015 Men's Asian Cup Tournament held in Australia. In other words, she has had a highly impressive career in football administration and is one of the most prominent examples of the way Australian women's sport was built and nurtured in a large part by gay women.

In 2019, Heather was asked to stand for election for the new board of Football Australia. It was an opportunity she felt she could not turn down. 'I had been part of the

Women Onside action to influence reform of Football Australia's governance and introduce the 40/40/20 gender principle in particular, so that we would see more women on the board,' she says. 'It was the first time in about ten years that there was going to be an election for the director positions. So when I was asked if I would accept the nomination by the Professional Footballers Australia [PFA] – the union representing professional footballers – I thought, well, I can't not walk the talk, given that I've been advocating for more women in leadership and on the board.'

However, as the election loomed, Heather noticed some health concerns that she couldn't ignore. For a few years she had been experiencing what felt like severe menstrual cramps, although she was more than ten years past menopause. It reached a point where she needed medical advice, and to her immense shock, Heather was diagnosed with stage four endometrial cancer.

After a hysteroscopy, followed by a hysterectomy, Heather was informed by her gynaecological surgeon that they had found malignant cells in the peritoneal washing, which meant she would require chemotherapy and possibly other follow-up treatment. 'I said, "That can't be right. I can't do this, I'm about to be elected to the board of Football Australia",' she tells me candidly.

'And the specialist said, "You have to make some decisions. You have to make some choices here. What is more important to you, your health or this position on the board?" I thought that was pretty brutal.'

Brutal as it was, Heather needed to make the decision. In the end, it was the advice of a close friend who was also living with cancer that helped her. 'Her attitude was to continue with the election process,' Heather says. 'And once I'm there at the table, I can decide what I want to do, whether or not it's going to be more stressful for me, whether or not I can cope with the business, whether or not it is a good distraction.'

The idea of focusing on something other than the treatment appealed to Heather and she thought she could manage it. 'At that stage, too, I had no idea how long I would have,' she says. 'Oncologists and specialists don't like to say you've got six months or twelve months, it's always a drip feed of information and treatment regimes. They couldn't say whether I'd have two years, three years, or what the survival rate is.'

So Heather took it on, balancing the tumultuous period of chemotherapy with taking on a new onerous role after a landslide victory and being appointed as Deputy Chair. Unfortunately, what began as a significant appointment, combined with a distraction from the shock of her cancer diagnosis, soon spiralled into a separate yet intersecting traumatic experience.

In the aftermath of the removal of the then coach of the Australian women's football team in 2019 – a unanimous decision by the board – Heather was hounded by the media to comment on the sacking. It was then that she made what she describes as an uncharacteristic 'error of judgement' when she spoke to a journalist who said he wanted to write about homophobia in football. His final article chose to focus on a few poorly chosen words relating to the former coach and largely ignored her broader commentary on homophobia.

'I should have had my phone hidden in a box somewhere and not sent private and confidential messages to a few people,' she says. 'I also spoke to the journalist about some comments that had been made and before I knew it, I was embroiled in legal complexities. The subsequent personal attacks against me were horrible and well beyond the point of being reasonable.'

It was the last thing Heather needed while going through such a stressful time in her personal life. She had made the decision not to tell many people about her cancer and treatment, as she felt it was something she wanted to keep private and didn't want people's perceptions about her to be influenced by the news. But it was a lot to take on at once and she found that period of her life extremely distressing. 'It has taken me a while to come to terms with it because I felt betrayed and that I was being forced into silence,' she says. 'I have a very strong network of colleagues, very protective, very supportive. And they remind me often of the perils of Twitter and speaking to journalists, regardless of whether it's on the record or not. I've learned from that, but it still doesn't dismiss the fact that I felt I was being bullied and persecuted in a range of ways.'

From there, things got worse, to the point that in February 2019, Heather decided to take a leave of absence from the board to allow her to focus on her health and her cancer treatment. 'I thought I could handle what was going on, but it just became so personal, abusive and vitriolic,' she says. 'And so attacking, on social media especially, that I had to just stop for my own sanity.'

During her time away from the board in 2019, she got well enough to attend her sixth Women's World Cup in France, which she had been looking forward to as a way to unwind and spend time with friends and long-time colleagues she'd met at previous World Cups. But even her presence there was construed as an issue, particularly after she had been obligated to issue a public apology to the former coach. 'I went as a spectator, like I've done at other World Cups, and yet people were tweeting about me being there,' she says. 'Apparently I'm so sick, I can't be on the board, but I can be at the World Cup in France, what's going on? Unfortunately, I also didn't get a lot of support from my fellow directors during that time.'

Heather felt like it was a constant uphill battle, dealing with her cancer treatment and balancing this difficult position on the board. But throughout 2020, she finally started to feel like she was getting into a rhythm. 'I thought I was doing okay,' she says. 'It was a nice distraction. But it was a huge responsibility and a hell of a lot of work. I would spend hours preparing for board meetings. I like to take my time reading through papers like the financial statements, but when you're dealing with very complex issues, it can be even more time-consuming. You have to ask the right questions as a director and understand what's going on in the business. I took that role very seriously. I think the diversion is important, but it was hard work at the same time.'

Just as she was finding the balance she needed and taking comfort in the duties, she was blindsided not once, but three times. In August 2020, Heather's ninety-year-old mother, who called herself Heather's number-one fan, had an unexpected fall. Within a week, the family agreed to their mother's wishes to let her go because her injuries were too much to bear. Heather spent the last forty-three hours with her mother. Her death was devastating for Heather – to lose someone so important and close to her in this period of her life was almost unbearable.

The next issue arose when Heather was in mandatory hotel quarantine for two weeks after she'd spent time in Canberra to be with her mother and family. She was told about a potential new director standing for election on the board. Heather had some questions about the candidate, who had been publicly critical of the board, the president and herself over the termination of the former coach. She put this to the chair of the nominations committee in order to find out more about the candidate's propriety for the role. 'Not long after I spoke to the other director, I was then subjected to what I would call a fairly vexatious claim of trying to interfere with the election of a director,' she says. 'But in fact, I was doing my job as a director by asking questions about the suitability of this potential new member and I was treated like I was a naughty little girl.'

It was at this point that the role began to feel like too much for her. It was no longer helping her to get over the traumatic experience of cancer treatment, but becoming an ongoing trauma of its own. At every turn, she felt she was being thwarted and the positives were no longer outweighing the negatives. 'I just felt so insulted and personally shamed,' she says. 'This was my character and my integrity that were being questioned, not to mention my duty as a director … I just felt ashamed, and I couldn't really say too much about cancer, I didn't want to use that as an excuse. I didn't want it to be used by other people to make me seem more vulnerable.'

At this stage, Heather was nearly ready to walk away from being a director and put the difficulties it caused behind her, but she persisted as she felt that she needed to fight the allegations for her own dignity and self-worth. The president of a state member association used a little-known clause within the *Corporations Act* to move a motion for Heather's removal from the board and the decision would require a vote of all members. There was no requirement to provide reasons for the motion. 'I spent the next two months outlining my case to the members, explaining my actions and trying to rationalise why I should remain on the board,' she says. 'I had terrific backing from my own personal support system as well as trusted colleagues in football.'

In February 2021, the vote was held and Heather lost by the smallest of margins, something she still struggles with, knowing that there were members who she believed were going to vote against the motion but chose to abstain rather than support her. It was a hurtful way to lose her position, but after giving herself a couple of days to sit with it, she began to feel relieved. It was finally over. 'The business of Football Australia, like any large organisation, is intense,' she says. 'It's demanding and it's voluntary ... Once I'd had some time to take it in, I just felt that I didn't need that anymore, I could focus on other things.'

The final blindsiding came when she visited her gynaecological surgeon for a routine check-up following her regular blood test and scans in July 2021. 'I was feeling pretty well, but I'd been to the doctor about a sore throat and she recommended I have another CT scan,' she says. 'The results were sent to the gyno surgeon and so he read them first and then he said, "Oh, dear, you've now got pulmonary metastasis." I kind of felt like he was washing his hands of me, saying there's nothing more he could do for me, just sending me back to the oncologist. I was stunned to say the least.'

It was a shock for Heather, who had been feeling healthy and finding more things in her life to look forward to and enjoy after her removal from the board. Most of all she dreaded the idea of having to undergo more chemotherapy. She had to see a new oncologist and was fortunate to find someone who was able to get the lesions in her lungs under control with the use of a progesterone treatment called Provera. 'I'm doing well, I feel well, I'm physically active,' she says. 'I do yoga a couple of times a week, I don't feel sick. I've just got these little lesions in my lungs that I need to keep under control. I just take one little pill every night and thankfully, so far, it's doing its job. The lesions aren't growing or spreading, some of them are hollowing out. Apparently, it's hard to even see that they're there.'

I am intrigued by Heather's pragmatic nature and how she has taken all these setbacks in her stride. I ask what her secret is, and she is characteristically upfront. 'I have a strong and powerful support group that I named The Posse,' she tells me. 'This group of fabulous women have protected me from further social media criticism, nurtured me, reminded me to put the phone away and helped keep me sane over the past five years. These are women who I trust, and I love dearly, because they said, "We will protect you, we will provide support for you".'

These friendships have fuelled Heather in both her professional and personal life, giving her a lifeline in the times of extreme stress, grief and difficulty. 'If I've been doubtful about something, I can just write a note and get all their responses,' she says. 'We have a group chat where we talk about all sorts of things, from commentary on the A-League Women's games to broader issues in the game, through to personal problems that we're facing. The Posse initially was there to help me with the anxiety of living with cancer, to be more careful with social media, and to help me rebuild my confidence. Some of them have also been through cancer, so we can compare notes about treatment or the uncertainty that we feel – it's an amazing group.'

For Heather – who had so many feelings of betrayal and a lack of trust in the difficult professional times she experienced – knowing that she has friends who have her back is absolutely key. 'They have a very broad, sweeping amount of expertise and experience, but above all what makes them special is the level-headedness and unconditional love for me and what I've done and the contributions that I've made to the game,' she says. 'They don't want to see me gone. They make me want to try and be ... what's that expression? A sparkling unicorn in a world of jackasses.'

Not long before her diagnosis, Heather had moved from Canberra, which she had called home for most of her adult life, to the Sunshine Coast hinterland and the beautiful property that she shares with her partner. While the remote location could have led to feelings of loneliness during her cancer treatment, instead she found it gave her the opportunity to stay connected with the people she chose to have in her life and provided privacy from those she did not.

'I think I always knew the kinds of friends that would want something from me for their own purpose, whether it was information or advice or an introduction to somebody,' she says. 'I didn't have to deal with any of that additional pressure. I just had my own little space. I did have friends come and stay during my treatment, good friends who I didn't mind seeing me without my hair!'

The ability to truly choose the people that she wanted to share this difficult part of her life with removed a lot of the burden Heather could have faced during her illness. Rather than being buried in requests to help, Heather was able to be discerning about who was part of this journey and draw genuine support from them. 'I spent decades working in sport and I think I can be more selective about who I choose to engage with in a meaningful way now that I have this kind of refuge up here,' she says. 'I was CEO of Capital Football for the last twelve years, and I ran Canberra United for almost ten years, so at the end of my career, there were literally thousands of people who knew me.'

The sheer scale of Heather's networks made it difficult to narrow down the people she brought along with her and kept in the loop, and the numbers don't seem small to those without the context of her career. 'In one of my discussions with my psychologist I said, "I'm only telling a handful of people about my situation, maybe thirty or forty people." She nearly spat out her tea!'

To Heather, it is not necessarily the number of people she shares personal information with that is important, but the quality of the friendship and support they provide. She prioritises family and those who have proved over the years that they are not fair-weather friends. Cancer has a habit of drawing out those who derive pleasure from being close to tragedy and feeling like they are involved or have the inside scoop on what is happening. Heather's distance and isolation from the place where she had spent most of her life allowed her to avoid both types of people and protect herself from the emotional harm they could cause.

'There are so many people who want to know how I'm going and I choose carefully about what I say to some people,' she says. 'If I was in Canberra going through the treatment, I don't think I would have had the same amount of peace, the same amount of privacy. And the same amount of rest that I needed during the treatment process. Now when I go back, I can choose whether or not to say I've got metastasis or I'm just doing okay, but still challenged. Because if one person knows and they see someone else and say, "Did you know Heather Reid's still got cancer?" suddenly it's out of my control.'

While stage four cancer is generally not considered curable, it doesn't necessarily mean an immediate death sentence. Heather does not know how much longer she will live, but for now, she is well and she is able to focus on enjoying her life.

'What I have to keep in mind is that everything I'm doing – from taking the Provera, to having regular acupuncture and taking Chinese herbs every day to keep my immune system strong, doing yoga and gardening, to seeing the psychologist and talking about it with people I love and trust – it's all contributing,' she says. 'I hope to live a long life. I'm reasonably financially okay, so I can do stuff like go on holidays and see my friends. My focus is to see as many women's football games as I can while I can, and just try to enjoy life as much as possible.'

The fact that Heather experienced a huge professional crisis while at the same time going through deep personal grief has given her a unique perspective on building a life after experiencing trauma. Most importantly, her experiences have helped her understand that she feels most fulfilled when she lives in ways that align with her values. This is easier said than done, but after many years of figuring it out, she now feels she has it sorted. Through this attitude and her relative isolation, she is able to choose to take part in projects that inspire her and allow her to make positive change. 'I'm continuing to give back,' she says. 'I am a leader in our sport. I read this terrific thing about leadership, and how it's not about leading from in front, it's about leading with others. And that's my style of leadership.'

Heather is on the board of an organisation called Women Onside, which aims 'to significantly improve engagement, access, opportunity and empowerment for all women involved in football.' Through this organisation, she has developed a mentoring program which provides women in the early stages of their careers access to experienced mentors who can help guide them as they make their way in this tough world.

'The work that I'm doing with the Onside Mentoring program is so rewarding for the mentees and the mentors, but also for me, seeing the growth of the mentees working with exceptional mentors in the last few years, that's what gives me satisfaction,' she says. 'For many women in sport, and particularly in the male-dominated football world, they just need someone to talk to, they need someone to help them with their goals, setting their expectations. That's what this mentoring program does.'

While Heather still finds distraction to be an important technique to help her get through the day, she now understands that the distraction can be more purposeful and doesn't need to be as stressful as the Football Australia board role she took on. It can be found in smaller things, closer to home, and in things that bring her joy.

'I do think the distraction is important for me,' she says. 'Some people find distraction in exercise, or in family. Some find it in meditation – I can't sit still, so I'm hopeless at meditation. My meditation is being in our bush garden and weeding and constructing things. I do a lot of outdoor stuff. When I can, when it's not too hard, that's my meditation – pulling out very large amounts of nasty weeds.'

What stays with Heather most of all from her experiences is the significance of trust in her life.

'Trust is really important,' she says. 'That's why The Posse is so important to me, I trust them implicitly. In the past, when I was giving lectures or presentations at conferences, I was somebody who always encouraged women to stand up when they see something that's wrong, whether it's discrimination, bias, homophobia – stand up, have the courage to speak the truth and be brave. But you can't really do that unless you have a support group that you can trust to back you. And it's the same with the cancer stuff. There's no need to feel you're alone with your anxiety or uncertainty.'

* * *

Heather's story and the wisdom she shares are particularly interesting to me because she comes from my world.

Although I have not experienced the same stresses she has on a professional level – in no small part because I do not have anywhere near her profile – I can relate to the trouble she has faced. I understand the difficulties of being a woman in sport and have had my own experiences of feeling like a 'naughty little girl' when I have done something that men in power have not liked. While this is not unique to women in sport – it is something that many opinionated women have faced in their professional and personal lives as an unfortunate symptom of living under the patriarchy – it is particularly prevalent in sport due to its history as a hotbed of traditional masculinity.

Women's sport in Australia has a long history of being built and run by gay women. Heather suggests when we speak that this was in part due to the fact that the gay women of those eras did not usually have the same level of family commitments as straight women. But in part it is also because of the safe haven they were able to create, and the joy they found in these communities meant that they wanted to give back. When mergers with male sporting bodies began to take place, there was a lot of discomfort from the men in power about lesbians. The women who were able to persist through these times to continue to work in sport were subjected to a great deal of homophobia. As a pioneer who helped move women's football from the amateur to the professional space – and a gay woman – Heather has experienced a great deal of discrimination, fear and gatekeeping, and this has been highly influential in the way she has learned to trust only those who have proved themselves trustworthy. With this backdrop, her focus on trust makes a lot of sense.

Heather's description of her relationship with The Posse is wonderful and I love the circle of trust she has created with these women. Adult friendship can be incredibly complex – we often don't get to see our friends as much as we would like and people's lives move at different paces and take them to different places, making it difficult to maintain friendships. While Heather's move to such a remote location could have left her feeling isolated, instead she was able to create a refuge for herself – away from people she did not trust – and built a community with people whose love and trust were unconditional.

Friendship is a subject that has always been a cause of anxiety in my life. I struggled with friendships as a child and a teenager and as an adult; I have always felt disconnected from other people. In most of my friendships, I feel that there is an imbalance and that I tend to like people more than they like me. Then my people-pleasing mode is activated and I feel the need to be extremely helpful so that people will be willing to have me around. This is part of the reason why I find that question 'What can I do to help?' so stressful. In the back of my mind, I worry that the person asking is only doing so out of obligation and if I take them up on the offer, they will surely get annoyed with me and drop the friendship at the soonest possible opportunity. It is always difficult to trace these anxieties back to find out where they have grown from, but I am sure that the way I was treated as a child and teenager – when I was told over and over again by friends and peers that I was annoying – contributed to this view of myself that I find so hard to shake. But after speaking with people who have been through cancer treatment or other kinds of trauma, I have learnt that I am not alone in fearing that I will drive away my friends by needing things from them. It is more common than I expected and knowing this has helped shape the way I respond to people dealing with traumatic events in their lives.

I have always felt that my approach to friendship, of having a variety of individual, unconnected friendships, rather than a set group who all hang out together, was a failure on my part. I thought friendship should look the way I saw it represented in popular culture and on social media – with big group trips away, weekends spent in each other's pockets and one big group chat which had all the answers. My discussion with Heather has forced me to reassess these feelings and to look at friendship differently. The Posse was gathered together to help her in a time of crisis and were women from different parts of the football world, joined together in love and support. They do not all live close together, nor do they have the opportunity to constantly spend time together. Their friendship is physically distant but emotionally close, and when they are in the same room, it is like no time has passed since they last saw each other. Most importantly, there is implicit trust, which is worth much more than simple proximity and seeing a person every day.

While I did not have a big group of friends to all hang out and cry with me and make cancer treatment into a party, like you might see in the movies, the friends I did have were there for me every step of the way. The fact that they are connected to me individually means that I have stronger links to each one, rather than the distance that a group can sometimes create between particular members.

These little strings tying me to each of my friends were like lifelines. Each of them provided different kinds of care and comfort. My friend Ana and I have a weekly ritual where we get together and watch old episodes of *Grey's Anatomy* – sometimes it takes us ages to actually start watching the show because we first catch up on each other's weeks over tea and salt-and-vinegar chips, falling into familiar rhythms, solving problems, listening and laughing. After which we turn on the television and spend the next few hours complaining about Owen Hunt, who is inarguably the world's worst television character. Having this comforting routine during the most difficult period of my life was so incredibly important.

My friend Alex and I connect most often while walking. We don't find time as much as we'd like, but she makes an effort to carve out time from her packed schedule and we roam the streets of our suburb – sometimes alone and sometimes with her dog and baby in tow. She was someone I could always talk to about my deepest fears during cancer because I didn't feel like I was burdening her with them. There were things that felt too hard to talk through with Shaun or my family because I didn't want to scare them or add to their worries. Having someone who was a step removed and so emotionally strong was such a relief in my darkest times.

I don't see my friend Kirsty nearly as much as I would like because she lives in the eastern suburbs of Sydney, while I live in the inner west. (For people outside of Sydney, I am aware that statement sounds ridiculous, but these are essentially different worlds.) Kirsty and I have been friends since the beginning of high school, closing in on thirty years. And while our friendship is sometimes the embodiment of that meme *Adult friendship is just saying 'We should catch up' every few months until you die*, whenever we do catch up, I get that feeling that no time has passed. Despite not being physically close throughout our adult lives, we have maintained the emotional connection and grown in the same direction.

My friends Jenn, Craig and Bec are even further away from me – none live in my city and we haven't all been in the same room at once since Jenn's wedding in 2019. But we talk every day and – like The Posse – our trust and support for each other are unconditional. A lot of the time, we talk about our shared love of netball or bond over silly jokes. But the way they rallied around me during my illness and made sure I never felt alone, even though they couldn't physically be there during my treatment, was astounding. They sent so many gifts that I had to yell at them for sending too many, which they ignored in a loving way.

I would love to spend more time with my friends Leanne and Amy – they live up the coast and every time I go to visit them, I come home feeling so fulfilled and happy. I have known Leanne since I was nineteen and we were both living in Canberra, where we connected through ultimate frisbee and a shared love of the music of indie women with guitars. When she met her partner, Amy, a few years later,

I gained a new friend and spending time with both of them brings me so much joy. Soon after finishing treatment, I took Pia up to Leanne and Amy's coastal city and we spent the most delightful weekend hanging out with them. It is a time I will always treasure.

Heather's story has friendship at its heart. I love that she had these amazing people in her life that allowed her to cope with trauma so well. It is a reminder of the importance of friendship, that having people outside of your family who you love and trust is vital and also incredibly joyful. It also forces me to reconsider my own relationship with the whole concept of friendship and understand that I am probably not as bad at making and maintaining friends as I have always thought. Just because my friendships do not necessarily look the way I envisioned adult friendship as a younger person does not make me unlovable or just not the kind of person that other people want to be friends with. After all these years, maybe I can finally let this idea of myself go.

It is hard to reframe these things that I have always believed about myself at my very core, but with the time, space and perspective to really reflect on my friendships and feel the love that echoes back at me from my friends – especially during difficult times – it is clear that I may not have as good a grasp on myself as I thought I did.

While in some ways that is a frightening thought – that the image of myself I held for so long is dissolving – it is also comforting. As I look for ways to move on and redefine myself in the wake of my trauma, letting go of these perceptions of myself that have only held me back feels liberating.

CHAPTER FIVE

Like I Used To

'I strongly felt that I needed to go on with life and not let trauma take me over.'

One thing that really surprised me about having a life-threatening illness was the incredible mundanity of it all. When you hear the words 'You have cancer' you expect the world to stand still. How is it that the earth can continue to turn when everything is falling apart?

When I first got the news, I halted everything. Fortunately, we were just coming out of a Covid lockdown and there was not a lot to halt, but one of the first phone calls I made was to my manager at work, explaining what had happened and that I needed to take some time off. He was instantly understanding and empathetic and I was able to take that time off with no issues at all – an experience that is unfortunately not universal for people who go through trauma.

I extended my time off when I learned that my first surgery had not completely removed the cancer and that cancer cells were found in my lymph nodes – which is known as local metastasis – so a second surgery would need to be done. However, after six weeks, my sick leave ran out and I felt the need to return to work. Without paid sick leave, there was no way we could continue paying our mortgage or doing all those things we had become accustomed to, like eating and having electricity.

To be honest, that was not the only factor which influenced my decision. I'm in the privileged position of having parents who could and would have given me the money I needed to take more time off work, if I had asked. But while I thought about asking a few times, I could never bring myself to do it. I had this idea of myself as someone who just deals with hard stuff and pushes through it, even while going through the worst time of her life. I didn't want to have to ask for help and sit at home, recovering; I wanted to be the person who takes it all in her stride and keeps on being a productive member of society. I hated the idea of letting anyone down so much that I went along to a work event the night after my first chemo treatment.

My hair had not yet fallen out, so I looked completely normal. Inside, I felt like hell. I spent the next few days feeling sick and awful after pushing myself too hard – and also feeling guilty because I was asked if I had taken any photos at the event for our website and I had not. Even though it wasn't something I had been asked to do, and it had taken all my energy just to get through the evening, I felt like I had not been productive enough.

The idea of productivity is an interesting one. There has been a lot of discussion around my generation's obsession with it – from bragging about the hours spent working long after officially clocking off for the day to attempts to monetise every hobby and turn leisure time into yet more work.

Writer Bridie Jabour offers up an interesting explanation for this in her book *Trivial Grievances*: 'We want our lives to mean something, and lots of us don't have religion or lifelong communities to feel tethered to anymore,' she writes. 'We have moved more to being defined by what we have achieved, even if what we have achieved is three ten-kilometre runs in a week.'[28]

Anne Helen Petersen's essay for *Buzzfeed* on the subject 'How Millennials Became the Burnout Generation' went viral when it was published in 2019 because it resonated so much with people my age who were feeling almost constantly overwhelmed. In discussing the inability to perform simple tasks in her life, she begins to understand the deeper issues behind it.

'Why can't I get this mundane stuff done?' she asks. 'Because I'm burned out. Why am I burned out? Because I've internalized the idea that I should be working all the time. Why have I internalized that idea? Because everything and everyone in my life has reinforced it – explicitly and implicitly – since I was young. Life has always been hard, but many millennials are unequipped to deal with the particular ways in which it's become hard for us.'[29]

She also notes the way us millennials think about work as part of our personality in a way that often was not the case for our parents' generation. The old mantra 'do what you love' has been absorbed by millennials over our whole lives. I remember my dad hating work for basically my whole life – it was somewhere he was compelled to go in order to get the money to live, but he certainly wasn't passionate about it or ever seemed to expect to be so. My mum loved her work – and still does – but I saw that relationship to work differently because she was a nurse – you expect people whose work involves saving lives on a daily basis to have a greater investment in their jobs. Hers is a true vocation, not just a job. But for the adults I knew who had office jobs – a love for work was not something I ever witnessed. As Petersen notes, that began to shift with the advent of the internet, both because work suddenly had the ability to take over our lives and the lines between on and off the clock became arbitrary and blurred, and because social media started showing us the curated lives we believed other people were leading.

'(Millennials) internalize the need to find employment that reflects well on their parents (steady, decently paying, recognisable as a "good job") that's also impressive to their peers (at a "cool" company) and fulfils what they've been told has been the end goal ... doing work that you're passionate about,' Petersen says.[29]

We wear our busy-ness as a badge of honour. Spend any time at all inside an office and you won't have to wait long to hear people trying to 'out-busy' each other. Outside of work, it creeps its way into hobbies that we have monetised into becoming side hustles, activities that we take our kids to, social events that keep on coming. The pandemic forced us to stop and grapple with the idea of not being busy, and it felt for a while like we had learned a lesson – that it is fine and even desirable to slow down and not be consumed by work and schedules – and life would become more settled in the long term. But in a post-pandemic world, every month seems to bring another wave – more employers determined to get their employees back to the office full-time, more activities for the kids who missed out during the multiple years of lockdowns, more social events because people are now aware how easily it could all be pulled out from under them, so we might as well celebrate now. If anything, the busy-ness lifestyle feels like it is even more prevalent than it was before.

Tim Kreider explored the culture of busy-ness for his *New York Times* story 'The Busy Trap' way back in 2012. He noted that the people who most often talked about being busy were not the people he necessarily expected to have such an affliction; it was not something he heard among healthcare workers or those working multiple minimum wage jobs to make ends meet.

'It's almost always people whose lamented busy-ness is purely self-imposed: work and obligations they've taken on voluntarily, classes and activities they've "encouraged" their kids to participate in,' he writes. 'They're busy because of their own ambition or drive or anxiety, because they're addicted to busy-ness and dread what they might have to face in its absence.'[30]

Perhaps it is precisely because we have now faced its absence that we have returned to busy-ness culture with a vengeance. I remember vividly the feeling of watching my Google calendar trickle away over the month of March 2020, as various plans and obligations were cancelled.

At first it was a novelty, one I welcomed as I looked forward to a short period of rest and relaxation. But as the time stretched on and the calendar got emptier, the absence began to feel like a gaping hole in my life – one that I was desperate, but not allowed, to fill.

Experiencing a serious illness off the back of two years being in and out of lockdown, of plans being made, cancelled, modified, rescheduled as we worked out how to live in a changed world affected the way I approached treatment and recovery, increasing the unease I felt about yet another period of being unproductive.

This combination of feeling a need to constantly achieve, of work and being productive forming part of my personality, and an urge to keep busy weighed on me as I lay there with no hair, feeling wretched after having poison pumped into my body regularly over six months. The feeling that was able to creep through the sickness and fatigue and numbness was guilt that I was not working to the best of my ability. And so I kept on pushing through, feeling a sense of pride when I was praised for my attitude to keep working during this time, tinged with yet more guilt because I knew I 'should' have been doing more.

I can now recognise that there were certainly times that I could and should have taken more time to rest and recover, and that I certainly did not need to feel guilty about my lack of productivity. But I also wonder if work provided a good and useful distraction that I needed to get me through that difficult time. Perhaps I was pushing through for the wrong reasons, and a little too hard, but having this outside purpose may also have given me the tools I needed to not drown in fear and despair.

The idea of work as a distraction and a coping mechanism is one I wanted to explore further. Research involving survivors of domestic violence[31] and childhood sexual abuse[32] found both groups were inclined to extreme productivity, including overworking behaviours. While work may not always be a healthy coping mechanism, it also seems like it may sometimes be the distraction needed to get through a difficult period and provide the opportunity to tread water for a while. I want to delve more into this idea and explore the ways in which work can be a refuge that may help with moving on in the long term.

Mel

I speak to Mel one afternoon – she is on a rare day off from work. Like me, Mel has long felt the need to be incredibly productive and she juggles multiple roles in event management and fashion. While she now has a good balance between work and home life, during times of trauma and recovery, she has buried herself deep in work.

Mel's troubles began slowly, almost imperceptibly. She was working in a busy event management job and was excited to be working at the same company as her cousin. They had grown up together and were close in age, so they enjoyed working together.

'We would always hang out growing up,' Mel says. 'We didn't actually live close to each other, but every school holidays we'd go to my grandparents' house and we'd hang out and spend heaps of time together. Our families have gone on holidays together and then as we got older, we'd go out together and remained very close.'

However, as she began spending more time with her cousin at work, Mel started to notice a change in her behaviour. Her cousin was drinking heavily and often relied on Mel to help her out of trouble. It came to a head while they were working together on a major event interstate. 'While we were working on the event, there were multiple instances in the evenings where she would call me to pick her up because she had been drinking or she'd be having a panic attack,' Mel says. 'I'd have to pick her up at 1 or 2 am, bring her back to the apartment that I was staying in and make sure she fell asleep at my place. Then she'd get an Uber back to her apartment in the morning and we'd both go off to work. Because she was family, obviously I'd do anything for her. But in the back of my mind, I just kept thinking, I'm trying to do my job. It started to feel controlling and I felt like I was being manipulated.'

Mel made it through the event relatively unscathed, but she continued to be concerned about her cousin. Reflecting now, she can see that she subconsciously began to distance herself a little in order to avoid the controlling influence she could see in their relationship. Both left the company they had been working at together in the months following the event and began new jobs and, as a result, they were not as close as they had been before. Then one day, Mel's cousin called her to tell her that she was going to rehab to attempt to recover from an alcohol addiction. 'I knew she was a very heavy drinker, but as a family member, I never really thought that she should go to rehab,' Mel says. 'I don't think that's a normal thing that happens. I've never experienced anyone going to rehab before or what that looks like. But I was definitely very supportive of her decision once she told me. I thought it would be a really good thing for her.'

Mel continued to be supportive and visited her cousin while she was in rehab to keep her company and reassure her that she was not alone. Only Mel, her partner and her cousin's immediate family knew where she was, so Mel wanted to make sure she had visitors and felt cared for. During those visits, she began to notice her cousin had developed a facial tic, which was explained away as a side effect of some of the medication she was on. 'I thought she was actually doing okay when I visited, beside the tics, but I found out later she was really struggling with this medication she was on,' Mel says. 'She'd previously shown signs of anxiety and depression, but this medication seemed to heighten those feelings and it started to really affect her life.'

After coming out of rehab, the symptoms seemed to only get worse over the course of the next few months. She developed extreme sensitivity to sound and became unable to take care of herself. 'You could really tell that it was impacting her life because she couldn't do normal things on a day-to-day basis,' Mel says. 'There were a lot of instances where she'd have to leave work early because she just couldn't handle it.'

With very few people having knowledge of the situation, a lot of the caring load fell to Mel. As she was also working close by to where her cousin lived, she would often have to leave her job to take her cousin home. It was during one of these times that her cousin began talking to Mel about her will. Over the next few months, the conversations tipped more and more into suicidal ideation, and Mel found herself having to regularly talk her cousin down. But amid the fear and concern, Mel also began to recognise the controlling and manipulative patterns that had emerged during their time working together.

'I felt trapped and I didn't know who to talk to or what to do as she would manipulate me and I started to feel like she was using these discussions to control me,' Mel says. 'I don't doubt that her suicidal feelings were real and serious, but there was also an element of powerplay and getting me to rush to her side.'

One day when they met for lunch, Mel's cousin told her that the time had come and that day would be her last. Mel still remembers the feeling of her blood running cold. 'I told her not to go through with whatever elaborate plan she had come up with in her head and I rushed back to my office to grab my things so I could spend the rest of my day basically babysitting her to keep her safe,' Mel says. 'But before I knew it, she ran away from me with the intention of suicide. She turned off all devices so we wouldn't be able to track her. I called the police and they started a search for her throughout the city. Two police officers were also stationed at her apartment and they tapped into CCTV security footage around where we had been and anywhere we thought she might go, as well as trying to triangulate her phone.'

Mel was beside herself, desperately trying to hold it together as she worked with police, kept her cousin's parents and sister in the loop and tried to figure out where her cousin might have run to. She struggled to keep waves of guilt at bay as she tried to think of what she could have done differently to prevent the situation from coming to this. 'Then she started taunting me and her family by turning her phone on and off, just enough to not get a read on her location,' Mel says. 'Those were the longest five hours of my life. The whole time I thought it was my fault, knowing that I hadn't kept a close enough eye on her at a time when she wanted to end her life.'

Eventually her cousin was found ten kilometres from where she had run away from Mel, highly intoxicated and injured from falling on her face. Bystanders called an ambulance and once her minor injuries from the fall were treated, she was put back into rehab.

Mel was understandably shaken and soon after began to experience PTSD symptoms. She felt incredibly guilty about everything that had occurred.

'I felt like it was my fault, for tipping her over the edge and letting her run away from me,' Mel says. 'I don't think I stopped crying that whole day. I've never had that level of emotion in my life. I felt like I was in pain from crying. I know some people in those situations dissociate and feel like they're just watching it happen, but that wasn't my experience. I *was* the situation, I was heavily involved in what happened.'

While Mel had not previously felt that she had a particularly close relationship with her parents, after this traumatic event, she craved connection with her mother and immediately called her in tears. 'The first thing I wanted to do was go see my mum,' she says. 'So I just got in my car and drove the forty minutes to my parents' place. As soon as I saw her, I just cried and explained exactly what happened. I never thought I'd be that kind of person at all.'

Her mum suggested that she should seek out counselling. 'For her to tell me that I should seriously consider seeing a psychologist was a huge breaking point for me, because I never thought that they would be open to that idea,' Mel says. 'I had actually already been seeing a psychologist before that, but I wasn't very open about that with them. The fact that they actually said that I should talk to someone because I needed help processing what happened was a big relationship shift for me and my mum and our bond that grew from that.'

Mel had been seeing her psychologist for almost two years at that stage, but with her parents' encouragement, she began to talk to her about what she had been through with her cousin. The psychologist recognised her PTSD symptoms and suggested a form of exposure therapy to help her process them. 'I had to recount the pivotal moments of that day, and I'd have to do it over and over again,' Mel recalls. 'There was a specific moment from that day that I'd have nightmares about. I couldn't sleep, I'd close my eyes and I felt like I was transported back there, I could see where I was standing, how I was feeling. My psychologist got me to describe that scenario to her, exactly as I remembered it. Then I'd have to say it again and add more detail in and repeat it and keep adding more detail every time. We'd essentially have a fifty-minute session, with me just constantly repeating this and divulging how I felt after every time.'

Throughout this period of trying to recover from the trauma, Mel turned to work for comfort and distraction. She also took the opportunity to make the move from her home in Sydney to Melbourne, which allowed her to put physical distance between herself and her trauma for a fresh start. 'It was during Covid, so I went from being in lockdown in Sydney, then when I moved down to Melbourne, I had to do the two weeks quarantine,' she says. 'I got out for a day and then Melbourne went into lockdown. So I was physically isolated and alone for a long time during my recovery – from June to November. But during that time, I was working.'

While Mel had moved to Melbourne primarily for university, she was also working two jobs in event management, so she had plenty to keep her busy during the long days in her new home. 'Weirdly, I think it was the best thing ever for me. I just needed something to use my brain,' she says. 'I was just working constantly and didn't even feel like it was a bad thing that I was in lockdown, though I couldn't physically go anywhere. I think that was probably the pivotal moment where I realised how purposeful work made me feel.'

During this time, she was also able to keep up her sessions with her psychologist over Zoom, which – together with the useful distraction of work – she found helped her stay grounded as she worked through her PTSD. 'There were multiple instances where my psychologist would ask what I thought I needed, if I needed to write down my feelings and work through them,' she says. 'But I was actually just so happy to work and not think about it all the time.'

Mel feels that in those early months, she was not ready to think too deeply about what happened to her. She could do the sessions with her psychologist and work through the symptoms she was experiencing, but outside of that, she needed to put the whole thing to the side until she was ready to try to understand it. 'Once I got through that period of time, I was like, wow, I can really process everything now. But until that point, I just strongly felt that I needed to try to go on with life and not let trauma take me over. I just needed to live a normal life. And I needed to fully use my brain to be able to do that.'

Mel now feels that she has recovered from her trauma. While the events of that day and the ramifications they caused will never leave her, she no longer experiences PTSD symptoms and she has been able to move on with her life. In this new phase, work still plays an important role, but it does not consume her the way it once did. 'I've definitely been taking care of myself more,' she says. 'I still work a crazy amount. But I think I'm more selective, and I'm really allowing myself to take time to have a break. I'm doing a lot more self-care things and doing more things for myself in general. That's really nice.'

The fresh start in Melbourne has also worked for Mel in the long term. In a post-lockdown world, she has been able to get out and explore her new home, make friends and settle into a new rhythm of life. 'I think I just feel more at home now … getting to know people I work with and making connections and friendships here has been so nice.'

These new connections have also helped her split from the past. Her job in Sydney was entangled in her relationship with her cousin – all the times she had to leave work early to care for her meant that everyone was aware of what had happened and her friends and family all knew the details of what she had been through.

'Coming into a new city where the people I meet have no idea what happened in the past means that I get to be the person that I want to be, rather than this damaged person that I was feeling like back at home,' she says. 'So many people I knew in Sydney were aware of what had happened and I just felt like – not treated differently – but like they had that awareness that kind of hung over everything. So it's definitely nice being new here. I feel more like myself.'

Although she no longer feels entangled in trauma, Mel can see that her life is different now and that she is a different person because of what she has been through. She is not better or worse for having experienced trauma; just different. This primarily shows itself in the way she forms connections with people. 'I definitely feel like there's a certain level of trust I have to feel when it comes to making new friends,' she says. 'I know who I like to have close by me and who I trust.'

She feels comfortable sharing her past trauma with the people that she trusts and also finds it important, because although she has moved on, there are still times when she feels triggered. 'I never know when something can be a trigger and if I go through that I can have a mood change straight away. So I make sure that my friends are aware, but it's not the same as it was back in Sydney. People are aware, but not always looking for the damage.'

The triggers may never disappear entirely, but they have been slowly dissipating and, most importantly, Mel feels equipped to deal with them and not spiral when they happen. She now understands what she needs to get through these times. 'I'm very much a person that needs to process things on my own,' she says. 'I'll take some time out by myself and have really good music playing, relax and breathe. Sometimes I'll find comfort in going for a walk, moving my body, being outside or driving myself to the beach – I've always loved being by the water.'

Mel feels privileged that she has been able to access counselling and connect with a psychologist who was able to provide therapy that really helped her through this difficult time. 'I'm really lucky – I know what works for me and I know the feelings are temporary, so I can get through it,' she says. 'To know that I'll make it out the other side when these things happen is really helpful.'

The most significant way that Mel has been changed by her trauma is that she now knows herself much more deeply than she did before. The process of going through counselling to find what she needed to recover, as well as moving to a new city and discovering the person she wanted to be when she emerged from under her trauma has compelled her to know who she is and feel content with herself. 'I've learned just how strong I actually am,' she says. 'For a really long time, not being able to feel like I could function and live a normal life because of the feelings I had was really difficult. But allowing myself to feel the emotion and knowing that what happened to me isn't normal, but it is normal to feel the way that I felt about it, were so important.'

She has also learned the value of asking for help – something that plagues many people going through trauma. This is a tough lesson, particularly for people who have always found their worth in productivity and what they can do for other people. 'I know I can be really stubborn and the way I help myself is being alone,' she says. 'But I also know that the people I have around me now are really here for me. They know that if I'm coming to them, it is a big deal for me.'

Mel's ability to be kind to herself has helped her to engage with other people who are facing difficult times. It's a feeling I recognise – these are hard conversations to have with no point of reference, but once you have faced trauma yourself, they feel easier to begin. 'I just always want people to know that their feelings are valid,' Mel says. 'Whatever you go through, there's always a way to process it, but it has to be in your own way. I think a lot of people obviously try and tell you how to move on, or what to do. But the only person that can truly do that is yourself.'

* * *

Talking to Mel has helped convince me to be more gentle with myself around my need for productivity and the way I pushed through with work while I was undergoing chemo. I like the way she speaks about the importance of distraction – it was something that Heather also talked about, and these reminders give me pause to consider the role that distraction played in my own ensnarement in trauma.

I bring it up with my psychologist at the cancer hospital one day, this idea that I have held onto for so long – that continuing with life pushed me into survival mode, which stopped me from processing what was happening and really feeling my emotions. 'I think going into survival mode was probably a really appropriate reaction,' she tells me. 'It's really hard to process something while you're going through it. If you hadn't had those distractions, you might have become overwhelmed with emotion and got stuck, not being able to do anything else.'

It's a different way to think about my reaction. For so long I have been caught up in the long-term effects – the unprocessed emotions that I'm sure are still simmering beneath the surface, waiting to swell up and overwhelm me – that I have not stopped to consider what a refusal to step into survival mode at the height of my trauma might have looked like.

What if I had felt all of my emotions as deeply and fully as I could? What if I had taken a year off work and become a full-time cancer patient and focused all my energy on that? What if I prioritised my treatment over the banality of parenting – of coaching my daughter's netball team, managing her cricket team, being the class parent at school? What if I had swept aside all these distractions and just collapsed into the heartache of it all?

Maybe I wouldn't be sitting here now, grappling with what it means to live after trauma. Perhaps I would have processed it all, made my way through the stages of grieving for the life I had before. Maybe I would be full of wisdom and instead of a book full of questions, I would write one full of answers. Maybe I would have it all figured out.

But what I think I understand now is that it is not always possible to live for the best long-term outcome. Sometimes what is best for you in the long run would be disastrous in the here and now. As Mel notes, working, studying and feeling productive all played a role in filling her time and occupying her brain when it was not yet ready to deal with her complex emotions. Staying busy allowed her to let those emotions creep in, bit by bit, in a controlled environment where she lay in wait, armed with the appropriate weapons to deal with them. Had she spent those months in lockdown alone with her thoughts and no distractions, she may have become consumed with emotions and unable to function.

For me, the option to let my whole world collapse was never really a viable one. While, in an ideal world, it might have been best for me to let everything go and feel all my emotions, I do not live in an ideal world. In my world, there are still bills that need to be paid, a child who needs to be cared for and volunteer roles that no-one else is going to do. And perhaps even in the long run, this approach might not have worked. Even if these outside influences had not shaped the way I felt I had to react and I had let my world collapse, who is to say that would have worked? Maybe I would still be sitting here broken, unable to put my life back together after letting it fall apart.

Writer James Colley published a story that stuck with me, where he spoke about the way his perspective on the song 'Cat's in the Cradle' changed since becoming a father. Like me, as he listened to that song ad nauseam growing up, he thought about what a terrible father the song's protagonist was.

'The message of the song is simple: it's about a parent who did not care enough about his child,' Colley writes.

'That parent then receives their comeuppance when the child is older and has no time for him.'[33]

It was only as Colley experienced his own despair as he left for work and his child clung to him, not wanting him to leave, that he realised that the 'terrible, neglectful father of "Cat's in the Cradle" who lives his life full of regret, abandoned by his family, was caught in the same system ... that was in place long before we were born, which will prevail long after we are gone.'

Life does not stand still for us to sit and watch our children grow up and it does not stand still while we experience traumatic events. It moves at its own constant, relentless pace and there is nowhere to hop off and just sit for a while and figure out how you feel about it all. Even if I had managed to opt out of all those distractions that swirled around me while I had cancer, others would have emerged.

Like Mel, I also sought out a fresh start during my recovery. It wasn't something I necessarily thought about consciously when I first began looking for a new job, but reflecting on it now, I could feel that awareness – just as Mel spoke about feeling at her job in Sydney – hanging over my workplace. My frustrations flip-flopped from being concerned that I was being treated differently by some colleagues to being upset that I was being treated as if everything was back to normal by others. I craved understanding from them, unfairly so because I could not even give it to myself – a recognition that things in my life had fundamentally shifted and I was not going to be the same person as before or work in the same way that I once did. I didn't feel like I could ever consciously choose to rest when I needed it because I wanted to live up to the expectations of who I was before, which meant always being switched on – even outside of work hours. On the other hand, I also felt unable to effectively use work as a distraction. There were days that I wanted to dive in and let the rhythms of the work take me over, but it felt impossible while I was surrounded by reminders of my old life.

Those feelings were never going to subside while I remained in the same place and so I began to look for other opportunities. My hair had grown back enough that I might have just had a short haircut and there were no physical indicators that I had once been sick – save for the tiny radiation tattoos that were easily covered. I could walk into a new workplace and no-one would need to know what had happened to me. So that is what I did. I said my goodbyes and my thankyous – for I was truly grateful for the opportunities and support I was given – and began my fresh start.

It was only after a couple of months that I started to feel uneasy. From the beginning of having cancer, I had always been open about it. I shared my story on social media – mostly because it helped me, but I later discovered it helped other people be more vigilant in their checks and advocate for themselves better with doctors. Now, I didn't have to tell anyone, but after being so open for so long, it felt like a weird kind of secrecy.

I also realised that being a cancer patient isn't something you can ever leave in the past – not just on an emotional level, but on a day-to-day scheduling level. My ongoing treatment plan involved follow-ups with three different specialists, annual ultrasounds and mammograms, a monthly injection to put me into menopause and a daily tablet to further suppress my hormones and prevent recurrence. It is a lot more involvement with the healthcare system than the average person – a healthcare system that does not care if you have to work and never provides any flexibility in appointment scheduling.

If I simply told my new managers that I had a doctor's appointment every time one of these cropped up, they would soon be wondering what on earth was wrong. So I decided I would start by telling them that I'd had cancer and these appointments would crop up from time to time and I would keep them in the loop and work my hours around them. They were immediately understanding and supportive – just as my previous workplace had been. Shortly afterward, I took a plunge and dyed my hair blue. That change was the impetus I needed to tell more people at work what I had been through. Every time someone commented on my hair, I got the opportunity to tell them what had happened in a way that wasn't sad or difficult.

'Thanks, I'm really loving it being so bright!' I'd say. 'I lost all my hair last year doing chemo, so when my hairdresser shaved it off for me, we made a plan that when it grew back, we'd dye it a fun colour!'

It was a great conversation starter and gave me the opportunity to frame it positively so people wouldn't feel sorry for me, but instead get to participate in my joy that all this was behind me and I got a fun hairstyle out of it. Once I started telling more people, I had some really good conversations, but I also realised there was a difference when people find out about a traumatic event that is behind you compared to the people who are there to experience you go through it. The awareness that hung over me at my previous workplace felt like a heavy woollen blanket that was stifling me as I tried to figure out whether I wanted to be treated exactly like I was before or if I wanted people to recognise I was a different person. This awareness was different somehow. It was lighter, more like a mosquito net drifting high above me so that I barely noticed it was there.

None of this is something I consciously understood or sought out in finding my fresh start, but listening to Mel's story and honestly reflecting on my feelings has given me a greater appreciation for what I led myself to. My relationship to work and productivity has shifted throughout the various stages of my recovery, and while I don't know if I have got that balance right yet – or if such a thing is even possible under capitalism – I feel like I now have a better understanding of how to take care of myself through both distraction and rest. It is a lesson that I will more consciously carry with me into the future.

CHAPTER SIX

You're the Voice

'Find a rainbow in every day.'

While I was still going through chemo, I was struck by the powerful urge to do *something*. Now that I knew what the experience of cancer was like, I felt like I had to help others who were experiencing it, no matter how small that help might be.

Sport has always been at the heart of both my personal and professional lives, so it seemed like a natural place to start. The McGrath Foundation is a charity started by Jane McGrath and her former Australian cricketer husband, Glenn. Jane died from breast cancer in 2008, but her legacy has lived on through the foundation, whose focus is providing breast care nurses to patients who could not otherwise access them. One of their fundraising initiatives is Pink Stumps Day, where individuals, sporting clubs and businesses can register to hold a social game of cricket to raise money. This seemed like something I could manage, even while in the depths of treatment.

In order to organise extra incentives for people to register and donate, I started contacting some of the professional athletes I knew from my years working as a sports journalist. Many of them had been in touch since they heard the news of my illness and had offered support. I asked them if they could donate any prizes of signed merchandise and they responded in kind. Before I knew it, packages were arriving multiple times a day with shirts, dresses, jerseys, bats and balls, all signed by some of Australia's best athletes. For every $10 donated to the fundraising page for the event, people would get one raffle ticket and could win one of these pieces of signed merchandise.

I was able to raise over $3000 for the McGrath Foundation, but unfortunately was not able to hold the cricket game in the end – being in the middle of a La Niña period, rain scuppered the plans for the match. Instead, I held the raffle at home and sent the prizes off around Australia to the winners.

While it was satisfying to raise some money, the disappointment that I didn't get to actually hold the event, combined with the fact that I had only been able to do something small, left me feeling empty. While I'd originally believed that even making a small contribution would help me feel better, once the reality of the smallness of what I had done hit me, I knew I needed to do something big.

It was the first time I realised the power of advocacy – not just for the cause itself, but for people who have been through something traumatic to process their own feelings. When I was diagnosed with cancer, I felt so small and ineffectual. My body had betrayed me and I had to put myself in the hands of the doctors and nurses and hope the treatments they had planned for me would save my life. There was nothing I could do to help myself. But by raising money and advocating for better care, I could do something for those who would come after me. Like Cher Horowitz, the iconic heroine of the movie *Clueless* giving her friend a makeover, it gave me 'a sense of control in a world full of chaos.'

The realisation made me curious about whether other people who have experienced trauma also feel this way. I have always thought of people who advocate for particular causes after their own traumatic experiences to have been doing it out of duty, a desire to protect other people from what they have been through, and I've assumed that it was also done with great personal sacrifice. But my own yearning to wrest back some control through fundraising and advocacy led me to think differently.

In her thesis *From Survivor to Advocate: The Therapeutic Benefits of Public Disclosure*, Katherine Infusino explores the therapeutic benefits of advocacy for survivors of sexual assault. Although only a small study, with three participants taking part, it is interesting to note that all three reported significant benefits from disclosing their experiences publicly and becoming advocates for the cause. One of the study participants notes that helping others through advocacy helped with feelings of shame and says, 'part of my rebuilt self-worth and rebuilt sense of community ... is that other people have benefited too.' She also believes that through disclosing her assault and helping others she 'felt a little bit of that power coming back.'[34]

Advocate Saxon Mullins was thrust almost instantaneously into the advocacy space when she appeared on a 2018 episode of the ABC current affairs show *Four Corners*, titled 'I am that girl'. Mullins gave up her anonymity to speak out about an incident in Sydney's Kings Cross, which had been the subject of a high-profile court case. In the years since, she has become the Director of Advocacy at Rape and Sexual Assault Research and Advocacy, a role that she has found unexpectedly healing.

In a story for *marie claire Australia*, she writes that the community she has found since becoming an advocate has been hugely important to her. 'They have helped me not only heal myself but to learn how to heal others with me.'[35]

Reading these stories makes me realise that this is a path I want to explore more. In my work as a sports journalist, I have come across some particularly special professional athletes who have gone down the advocacy route and used their public platforms to raise money and awareness for causes close to them. I want to learn more about why they have started down this path, and if it has brought healing to their own lives.

Amy and Molly

As a netball fan, I have long been enamoured with Amy Parmenter. It's hard not to be. She plays wing defence, which anyone with a passing knowledge of netball understands is the most criminally underrated position. Wing defences are hardworking and often the heart and soul of the team. They hold things together, but their work often goes unnoticed and unacknowledged, while the flashier positions on court take the credit.

Amy burst onto the scene in 2019 in her debut season for Giants Netball in the Suncorp Super Netball competition, winning the league's rookie of the year award. A bright future beckoned, and not long after she made a name for herself on the court, she stepped up her work off the court by committing more time and energy into the Tie Dye Project, a fundraising initiative she developed with her sisters in 2017. Amy's mother had taught her daughters to tie-dye as children, and after her death from mesothelioma in 2013, they decided to use those skills to raise money for cancer charities.

In 2018, soon after Amy first began training with the Giants as a junior member of the squad, she met Molly Croft at the Children's Hospital at Westmead. Amy was immediately impressed by Molly and speaking to her, it's not hard to understand why.

'I was diagnosed on my twelfth birthday with osteosarcoma,' Molly tells me. 'I live in Dubbo [five hours north-west of Sydney], so pretty much overnight, I was sent down to Sydney and I didn't really go home for about a year.'

Their meeting came during a radiothon for the hospital. The hospital staff knew Molly well by then and had realised that she loved netball. So when Amy and fellow netballers Kiera Austin and Sophie Garbin came in, they made sure Molly had the opportunity to meet them. 'Someone took me over and I think we spent about twenty minutes together,' Molly says. 'It wasn't too long. Ames and I and all the girls – well, I think we connected! I don't really know if I said too much. I think I just laughed at everything Amy said for the majority of it.'

After the group went their separate ways, Molly's parents took her to the hospital cafe. They were chatting about the day and the excitement of meeting the netballers when Amy came back in. 'She just said to me, "Mol, you've really touched my heart." And she actually took off her Giants jacket and gave it to me and gave Mum her number. And the rest is history. She's become like a big sister to me,' recalls Molly, smiling.

Amy's history with fundraising had started years earlier, stemming from the powerlessness she felt when her mum was sick. 'I just remember having this feeling of being so helpless, like I just couldn't do anything,' she says. 'I feel like it's such a common feeling for people whose family are going through things and there's nothing you can do to make it better.'

Her first venture was cutting off her ponytail to raise money for the Cancer Council when she was just fifteen years old. 'I felt like I was making a little tiny difference,' she says. 'Even if it wasn't going to help Mum, it was going to help those diagnosed later on or going through cancer treatment. And I thought, "I'll just get stuck into it, see what we can do."'

Amy had just started playing in the lower divisions of the Netball NSW Metro League – a competition far removed from the level she plays at today – but word spread through the netball community about her initiative and before she knew it, four members of the Australian Diamonds, the national netball team, were planning to come down and take part in the event. Amy's idol, Gabi Simpson – who was also a wing defence from Amy's home association of Randwick – was the one to cut off her ponytail, a special moment for the young netballer. The involvement of the Diamonds, who she looked up to so much, taught her a valuable lesson about making a difference that she has taken into her own career.

'It made me think, if I'm going to be a professional athlete, I need to know what it's all about, it's not just about throwing a ball around,' she says. 'It's about showing up for those fifteen-year-old girls that you don't know. Those netballers had such a big impact on me. I was beside myself that they cared enough to come along.'

This venture created a little spark in Amy that would go on to become the roaring fire that is the Tie Dye Project. It stoked in her a love for fundraising that would continue throughout her life. 'It was such an emotional and hard time for my whole family,' she says. 'But it was one of the first times I'd felt that little hole in my heart get a tiny bit smaller; I felt a little bit of happiness in a time that was really, really hard. And I think from there, it taught me that I had such a passion for fundraising and for bringing communities together for a common purpose.'

Molly too found a sense of peace and belonging through fundraising. When she returned to Dubbo after her long stint in hospital, she founded Molly's Mission. She first raised money for Ronald McDonald House. 'I know that I have been left on this earth for a reason,' she says. 'When I started fundraising, I was just thinking about all the love and support I got in hospital and I wanted to pay it forward. That's the true reason why I believe I'm still here.'

The small fundraising event she held in her home town wildly exceeded her aim of raising a few thousand dollars and she ended up with over $190,000 to donate to the place that had been a home away from home while she was sick. 'Ever since then I just fell in love with doing it,' she says. 'I was lucky enough to go to a Barack Obama speech recently and one of the last questions he was asked was, "What's your advice for young people today?" He said that his advice is that it doesn't matter if you don't know what you want to be, as long as you know what you want to do. And that really clicked. As soon as I had recovered from my treatment, I knew that what I wanted to do was to fundraise and create awareness for sarcoma.'

Once these two powerhouses came together, the Tie Dye Project really took off. Through Molly, Amy found the direction she had been subconsciously looking for to create a big impact. 'I had been doing the Tie Dye Project for a few years before I met Mol, but it wasn't anything too big,' she says. 'I feel like as soon as Mol jumped on board, it sort of exploded and became a lot more. I think our reach really grew and we had a bit more of a purpose and we were a lot more specific with what we were going to raise money for. The first few years it was really small. I'd just done it because it was a cool way of raising money. I'd do it with my sisters and it brought my family together a little bit. And then Mol jumped on board and suddenly we were really moving.'

Both Amy and Molly are incredibly proud of the work they have done to date. Sarcoma is the leading cause of cancer deaths for fourteen to twenty-four-year-olds, and the treatment for this kind of cancer has not changed much in forty years. Amy and Molly became aware of a clinical trial being conducted into a new type of immunotherapy known as CAR T-cell therapy – the same treatment that Greg was hoping to access for multiple myeloma – which has been hailed as the possible silver bullet for a number of cancers. In November 2022, Amy travelled to Dubbo for a very special tie-dye session. Over two days, all of

Amy's teammates at the Giants, along with crosstown rivals the NSW Swifts and Kiera Austin – who was with Amy when she first met Molly and has remained part of the Tie Dye Project even after changing clubs to play in Melbourne – set up camp under huge marquees and tie-dyed everything they could get their hands on. They were able to dye thousands of t-shirts, hats and netball bibs. Once these went on sale, they were quickly snapped up, raising over $100,000 for the CAR T-cell therapy clinical trial with just that one initiative. Molly is still struck by how significant that weekend was.

'If you put it in an NRL context, I don't think I've ever seen rival teams come together like that for one cause,' she says. 'The fact that they put aside their rivalry and they came together to support sarcoma – something so close to my heart – is really special. The Tie Dye Project is heavily volunteer based, so without the netball community and Amy's friends and my friends, the Tie Dye Project would be nothing. They are the building blocks – we couldn't do it without community.'

Together with the Kids' Cancer Project, they raised $250,000 over two years that was donated to this clinical trial.

'They've now been able to get $2.2 million of government funding, which will support the project for the next five years,' Amy says. 'And to think we were just tie dying in the backyard! To know that all the people who have shown up and tie-dyed over the weekends can be a part of something so massive, is really amazing.'

They also love the results of their work being so immediately evident. 'Something I'm really proud of with us is that wherever the money goes, I feel like we can tell everyone the difference that they're making, they can see the doctors and the researchers that are getting employed from the money,' Amy says.

'I was lucky enough recently to go to the lab where the scientists who we're funding and the equipment that we have funded, is actually being worked on and I got to meet the scientists, which was so cool,' says Molly. 'I got to look at the CAR T-Cells through a microscope working on two different types of cancer. I think what's also really amazing about the Tie Dye Project is we are lucky enough to raise such large amounts of money and 100 per cent of whatever we make goes toward the research and whatever we're fundraising for, which is something really special in itself too.'

As the Tie Dye Project has gained momentum, the awareness around it has grown. When Amy was first selected as part of the Australian Diamonds squad, the team was keen to become involved, and she found herself leading tie-dying sessions with Australia's greatest netballers while preparing to make her debut. It was a surreal experience. 'I just had a moment when that was happening where I was like, this is so cool that my netball heroes, and also my rivals, are all coming together for this common cause,' she says.

Through netball, Amy has also been able to inspire the next generation, not just with her skills on the court, but with her advocacy. She has been particularly impressed with Swifts player Sophie Fawns, who has become an advocate for ovarian cancer research after losing her mother to the disease.

While Amy initially had to steel herself before watching a video Sophie had been a part of to raise money for an early detection test for ovarian cancer, once she was able to watch it, she was incredibly proud of the young player. 'It took me a while to watch, if I'm being honest. I knew it would be a bit close to home,' she says. 'But when I watched it, it just made me beam. She's only nineteen and she's using her voice and her platform to make a difference. I just thought, that's literally what it's all about. It's such a privilege to have a platform and to have a space where people care what you think, just because you throw a ball around. We should be using that for something good.'

While Amy realises it will not be every athlete's desire to be an advocate, she is immensely proud that her decision to do so has spoken to other young netballers. 'I think it's so powerful what sport can do to drive change,' she says. 'It's something I'm really grateful to be able to do, because I didn't realise that I would have the ability to do that as a netballer. And hopefully it means that other girls coming through, like Sophie, will do it too if they want to.'

When I ask Amy and Molly where they want to take the Tie Dye Project next, they are reflective, but I can see the spark in both their eyes. Molly takes the lead with answering and Amy leans back in her seat, watching her young friend with joy as she speaks about their project with such passion. 'I think that the Barack Obama quote is very on brand with us right now,' Molly says. 'Because our vision is that we want to become Australia's most recognised charity for promoting grassroots awareness of sarcoma. But I guess that's more what we want to do. I really don't know what we want to be at the moment.'

She takes a moment to think, smiling at Amy and considering her words. 'We're at the point where we don't know how the Tie Dye Project is going to go. I think every day is a new learning block for us. We're terrible with emails and we're very not professional in any way. But I think what makes us really special is that we are just two girls wanting to create a bit of good in this world. I feel so lucky that I've been able to touch Ames and now through her profile, we're able to work together to create that good.'

The motto of the Tie Dye Project is 'find a rainbow in every day' – a sentiment that stems from Molly's time in hospital, where she would talk to her parents at the end of each day about something that made her smile. For Molly and Amy, the cause itself has become their rainbow as they change the lives of sick children and families and fight for a better future.

Sophie

Hearing Amy and Molly's story was so powerful that I feel like I can dig deeper and find more wisdom in this area from Sophie Fawns, who Amy was so proud to have inspired. I first met Sophie in 2022 when she made the move to Sydney from the regional town of Wagga Wagga to play for the NSW Swifts in the Super Netball and to start studying at the University of New South Wales, where I happened to be working at the time. Sophie joined the university's elite athlete program and I decided to write a story about her first year as a professional athlete for UNSW's news platform.[36]

The story tracked her journey over the year, so we spoke multiple times and I followed her career closely, attending a number of her games and travelling down to Victoria to watch her play in the Australian Netball Championships, a second-tier competition, when the professional league had finished its season.

I was drawn to Sophie's story in part because of the cancer connection. I was just returning to work and still going through my cancer treatment. Sophie's mother died from ovarian cancer in November 2021, soon after my diagnosis, and Sophie was still in the early stages of processing her grief when she moved to Sydney.

'It was really tough,' she says. 'I was supposed to go up for our preseason right after my HSC [Higher School Certificate] finished, but I didn't end up finishing my HSC. The Swifts were really supportive of it and they said come up when you're ready. So seven weeks later, we placed Mum in the temple and I just decided to move to Sydney. I thought, I want to start and this is what Mum would want me to do as well.'

It had been a tumultuous time in her life – juggling her final year of school with increasing netball commitments, supporting her mum as she got sicker and dealing with Covid lockdowns and restrictions.

'In 2020, Dad and I were always allowed to go with Mum for her treatment and scans,' she says. 'She had to go in alone but we could still come and sit outside the building.

But then in 2021 when everyone was in lockdown, we weren't allowed to go with her anymore. At the start of the year, I'd stay for three weeks at a time and do all the treatment with her up in Sydney and then after we went into lockdown in August, I was stuck in Wagga.'

Sophie's mum, Maureen, had been undergoing various treatments since her diagnosis in 2019, when Sophie was just fifteen years old. A routine surgery that Maureen had been putting off due to being busy discovered a single cancer cell. From there, she was rushed into chemotherapy. 'When anyone really hears the word cancer, obviously there's a lot of fear and you think of the worst all the time, but Mum was always very positive,' Sophie says. 'Whenever my sisters or I cried she'd always tell us to remain positive.'

After Maureen completed eight rounds of chemotherapy, she went for a review with her oncologist and discovered that the treatment had not worked; the cancer had kept growing and spreading. The next step was a clinical trial.

'There were three trials available for ovarian cancer and she didn't qualify for two, but there was one that she qualified for, so she started doing that, which was a twelve-month process,' Sophie says. 'Her treatment was going really well for ten months, and then suddenly it stopped working. She had a check-up every three or four months and at the ten-month mark they'd found she was doing really well so they kept doing it for another two months. Then when she had her twelve-month scan they found out that the cancer had spread all across her body.'

Maureen was put on yet another new treatment, but the doctors warned her that it was unlikely to work. 'In August, she had her scan before she started the new treatment,' Sophie says. 'Dad found out then that she was only going to have a few months to live but Mum never wanted to know and they never told us kids.'

In the early stages of her grief, Sophie struggled with regrets that she had spent some of that precious last time seeing friends, studying or playing netball instead of spending every waking minute with her mum, as she was unaware that their time together would be so short. But with time to reflect, she is able to be kinder to herself. 'At the end of the day, Mum never would have wanted us to stay home with her,' she says. 'She would want us to keep doing what we were doing and live normal lives.'

Sophie originally moved to Sydney after being named as a training partner for the Swifts. She was expecting to train a few times a week with the squad and focus on her university studies. But while Sophie was sitting on the bench during the first game of the season, Sam Wallace, the team's star goal shooter, ruptured her anterior cruciate ligament and was immediately sidelined for the rest of the season. Before Sophie knew it, she was catapulted into the team as a permanent replacement player – a role that involved much more intensive training and travel all over Australia for matches.

'There were a lot of emotions when Sammy got injured,' she says. 'But she was so supportive of me. She came up to me and said if I get the opportunity to take it with both hands. She was just so happy for me. I think that made it so much easier, I wanted to do her proud as well.'

It was a busy time, but Sophie welcomed the diversion and believes it helped her process her grief. 'I think netball was such a great way to keep me occupied, I just loved going in every day,' she says. 'And eventually it became not even about that. At the very beginning, it was a bit of a distraction. Whereas after a while, I realised I just wanted to be there.'

The times she has found it hardest over the years since Maureen's death were moments of heightened emotion. Competing at the Australian Netball Championships in 2022, she suffered a crisis of confidence and began putting too much pressure on herself to perform. 'On the first day when those emotions hit, I was like, "Oh my god, I just wish my mum was here",' she says. 'Looking up and seeing my dad sitting alone in the crowd was a bit hard.'

In the time since her mother's death, Sophie has grown and matured. She has completed a second season as a professional netballer and although she had less time on the court in her second season – due to the recruitment of an experienced player to cover the ongoing loss of Sam Wallace – she played a key role, often coming on court in clutch moments and scoring the goals her team needed. It was after both a last second win in the preliminary final in which Sophie scored the winning goal and an extra time, one-goal loss in the grand final that she felt the absence of her mum most acutely.

'I feel like this year is a lot different to last year,' she says. 'I've processed everything a lot more. So it's a lot less looking into the crowd and wondering where Mum is. But in those big moments like the grand final, I just wished that Mum was there and that she could have seen it. Even leading into the grand final, I was so anxious, so nervous, and all I could think was, "Oh my gosh, all I want to do is talk to my mum." She would have known exactly what to say.'

In those moments, Sophie has found the support of her teammates is what gets her through the hard and emotional times. She is now living with three of her fellow Swifts and in her team she has found a family. 'On court, in those big moments you're not really thinking until the game ends,' she says. 'So it hits all at once, but in those moments, I just go up to my teammates and give them a hug. It's not even me having to say I miss my mum – they just know and they say exactly what I need to hear. Maddy Proud [Sophie's captain at the Swifts] came up to me straight after the semifinal and said, "Your mum would be so proud." Little things like that are so special – even in the very high and the very low times for everyone, they still know and they're still saying she would be so proud.'

But like Amy and Molly, Sophie has also found peace and a calling of sorts in advocacy. Soon after Maureen's death, she set up a fundraising page in memory of her mother to raise money for the Ovarian Cancer Research Foundation. When we spoke for my story at UNSW, she was interested in doing more in this area, so as part of the story, we visited the Gynaecological Cancer Research Group, headed by Professor Caroline Ford, at UNSW. Professor Ford took us on a tour of her lab, introduced us to her team and showed us some of the groundbreaking work they are doing in the development of an early detection test for ovarian cancer.

During the tour, Professor Ford spoke about the group's partnership with fashion brand Camilla and Marc – a company headed by a brother and sister who lost their own mother to ovarian cancer when they were children –

and asked Sophie if she would be interested in getting involved with one of their fundraising campaigns. 'I was lucky enough that Professor Ford gave my email to Camilla and Marc,' she says. 'They reached out to me and asked if I could be part of this short documentary that they were making, to help raise funds for the [2023] campaign.'

Camilla and Marc put together four short documentaries featuring different people who had been affected by ovarian cancer – from people living with cancer to those who had lost family members to the disease. Sophie and her sisters got an opportunity to share their mum's story and, in doing so, raise awareness and funds for ovarian cancer research at the Gynaecological Cancer Research Group.

'We felt really privileged,' Sophie says. 'It was very special to be able to share that moment with my sisters. Obviously, we've never really done anything like that before. On the day, as exciting as it was, it was still sad and I was thinking, oh, I wish our whole family could be here for this. But the overwhelming feeling was excitement and pride that we got to be a part of something so special.'

Once the interviewers delved into the details of Maureen's illness and treatment, Sophie felt the wave of emotions start to build under her. 'At the start of the day, it was obviously very exciting, getting our hair and makeup done,' she says. 'But then when they started doing the interviews, it became a lot more real about why we were doing it, the reason for it. It was quite upsetting once we began, but being able to do it with my sisters, and having the support of our dad who came along to watch as well, was really nice.'

Once the campaign went public and the documentary was released, the wave of emotions began to shift and climb – sometimes in unexpected ways. 'At first, I felt very special that I was able to share Mum's story and our family's story, and that it was helping people educate themselves a bit more on this disease,' she says. 'But after a while I started to feel quite angry at times. It really hit me that ovarian cancer is researched so little and it frustrated me that people knew nothing about the symptoms and the statistics because there's just so little information out there about it.'

The theme of the campaign was 'Women deserve better' and Sophie began to feel this very deeply as she encountered reactions from people who knew very little about ovarian cancer and were shocked to learn about the lack of effective treatments and early detection tests. 'I felt like when the video was released, I just wanted it to be shared everywhere, so that people can educate themselves and understand what ovarian cancer is, and how they can help,' she says. 'A lot of people reached out to me saying they were so glad that they've been able to see this video because they didn't even know ovarian cancer was a thing. I think it helps that I've got a bit of a platform to get people to watch as well.'

Since her first steps into the advocacy space, Sophie has quietly taken inspiration from Amy Parmenter and was thrilled to be involved in the tie-dying weekend in Dubbo in late 2022. 'I think she's so inspiring, she's doing exactly what I want to do,' Sophie says. 'A lot of people look up to her because she's really built something off the court. But she's been able to bring it onto the court as well and use her position as a netballer for better, to spread awareness about sarcoma. At the tie-dye camp in Dubbo, all the volunteers were netballers, friends and family, all coming together to tie-dye shirts, so they can be sold and raise money for this really important cause.'

Sophie also admires the way Amy takes a holistic approach to the work she does – she is not only raising funds, but empowering people with knowledge. 'It's really special to see that she's bringing together communities, not just from netball, but we're able to interact with other people and there's lots of education about it,' Sophie says.

Sophie hopes she can make her own impact within the netball community and educate the majority female fanbase about ovarian cancer. 'The netball community has been so great,' she says. 'I think everyone just wants to help and we've seen the way they get behind the Tie Dye Project. That's what I aspire to with ovarian cancer.'

Importantly, Sophie feels that these steps into advocacy have been healing and have helped her process her grief. The powerlessness that Amy spoke about affected Sophie deeply as well, particularly when she wasn't able to accompany her mum to treatment anymore. Having a platform and using it to help change the fates of countless future women has been a way of taking back her power. It is what Sophie believes her mum would be doing if she had survived.

'When my mum was going through her treatment, she didn't really want people to know that she was sick,' she says. 'But she was always such a strong woman and advocated for what she wanted and what she believed in. My sisters and I have been able to grow up and watch her be that strong role model, so that now when it's our turn to talk about something we're passionate about, we're really putting our foot down. I love being able to spread awareness about ovarian cancer. I love when people ask me questions. It's also inspired me to do a bit more research into it so I can help educate other people about it when they ask me.'

It has been an emotional couple of years for the young athlete, but she has found her own path through them as she lives and plays for her mum, and not without her. Her strength has shone through as she has found a way to remember Maureen while also fighting to ensure other people will not have the same experience. Above all, she has found joy in life and although it is different to the joy she felt before her mum was sick, it is powerful in its own way.

'My mum would have hated it if I sat at home and sulked,' she says. 'When I think back, moving to Sydney was honestly one of the best decisions ever. I've got things outside of netball that I can do, I've made new friends. I can do these things and still live my life. And of course, something really traumatic has happened to me in terms of losing my mother at such a young age. But it changed my perspective on life so much, it changed me as a person. As crappy as it is, I wouldn't be the person I am today without those experiences. Obviously, I'd rather have my mum here, but I like the person I've become. I've learned that you actually don't have that much time and you shouldn't wait another day to do the things you want to do. You really should live your life to the fullest because you genuinely have no idea when it's going to end.'

* * *

Talking to Amy, Molly and Sophie helped me to understand and rationalise my own desires to find healing through advocacy. I have great admiration for all three of them, who are still so young and have found a way to turn their pain into good in the world. While Molly and Sophie have stayed close to the causes that originally affected them, I am particularly interested in the direction Amy has taken. Meeting Molly changed her trajectory and in this special young person, she has found the focus she needed to bring to her advocacy. While the tie-dying still provides the connection to and the memory of her mother, she has been able to find a cause for which she can make real change and that has deep ties to her community.

I think one of the reasons I have felt unfulfilled by my small forays into advocacy is a disconnect that I feel to breast cancer as a cause. Years before my diagnosis, when I did not really know anyone who had been through any kind of cancer, I felt frustrated by the almost constant attention breast cancer seemed to receive over other cancers and illnesses. Instead of running the Mother's Day Classic fun run one year, which raises money for breast cancer research, I chose to do my own run and donate money to ovarian cancer research, because I felt so strongly that breast cancer did not need more money.

When I was diagnosed, the memory of that decision haunted me for a while. I am not a religious person or a great believer in fate or karma, but I felt uncomfortable, thinking maybe I deserved this illness because of the way I had downplayed it in my mind and made a conscious choice not to contribute money toward it. Logically, I knew this did not make sense, but it was something that has stayed hidden in the corners of my mind and occasionally edges its way into my consciousness, even after my recovery.

In *The Undying: A Meditation on Modern Illness*, Anne Boyer reflects on the breast cancer marketing machine and her own discomfort. 'Every month is Pinktober when you have breast cancer and every actual October is a season in hell,' she writes. 'The world is blood pink with respectability politics, as if anyone who dies of breast cancer has died of a bad attitude or eating a sausage or not trusting the word of a junior oncologist.'[37]

Boyer writes about the co-opting of breast cancer by corporate interests, who by 1996 viewed it as a 'hot' cause, with pink ribbons adorning merchandise all over the world, used as a way to sell more to people who want to believe they are helping the sick. She writes about breast cancer charities in the United States whose CEOs are paid salaries of close to half a million dollars each year. Boyer tells the story of an activist, known by her online persona Coopdizzle, who died in December 2016. Coopdizzle fought for recognition and meaningful help for people with stage four breast cancer and against the culture of corporate 'awareness'. There is a pinned post on her Facebook page that Boyer references that particularly takes aim at the world's largest breast cancer charity, Susan G. Komen for the Cure.

'October is the best and worst month for me and my stage 4 sisters,' Coopdizzle wrote. 'The Pink ribbon stuff. First, it's not about THE ribbon. It's about the Komen. It's about the fact that when the REAL Susan passed from metastatic breast cancer, her sister said she would help find a cure. Thirty years later, we are no better off; in fact, it's gotten a bit worse. SGK only donates a very small amount to the research of terminal breast cancer. They shove us under the rug and act like we aren't real. They profit off your donations and have mansions and very nice cars.'[38]

In *The Undying*, I found a language that helped me understand the ways in which I did not feel part of the 'breast cancer community'. The detachment I feel is not with other people who have had breast cancer, but that the entire cause has been taken away from us. There is a forced disconnect as other people put themselves between us and our experiences, people who want to take the easy option and slap a pink ribbon on a product and sell it, sometimes donating a small amount to a breast cancer charity and boosting their own bottom line as they do so, other times not donating a cent. They want to hear our voices only when we are inspirational, positive and aligned with their strategies.

I know, of course, that there are people doing excellent work for the breast cancer cause – who are raising funds for good and meaningful things, like better care, improved treatments and research into causes and cures. But they have become obscured by this pink marketing machine that only seems concerned with 'raising awareness', which does nothing to support people who have been diagnosed with cancer.

The Breast Cancer Action group in the United States started the 'Think Before You Pink' campaign in 2002 to push back against this kind of marketing – particularly what they have called 'pinkwashing' in which companies 'who, while pretending to care about women and breast cancer, continue to spread misinformation, manufacture products that actually increase a person's risk for breast cancer, work to lower regulatory standards, and much more, all while raising millions to feed their own bottom line.'[39]

At the heart of this issue is the sexualised nature of the illness – it is an area of women's health that has been heavily researched and funded in part because of the appeal of breasts themselves. How often have you seen campaigns for breast cancer awareness urging you to 'save the boobies' or 'save the tatas'? They are everywhere, especially in October, and they usually feature plenty of imagery of breasts – often disembodied or without the face of the person visible. The message those of us who have had breast cancer receive is that it is our breasts that are worth saving, not us. For many people with breast cancer, saving their breasts was not an option and they have had mastectomies that have left one or both sides of their chests flat – a procedure that is life-saving, but is not often talked about amid the pink celebrations.

In Australia, the not-for-profit campaign group Collective Shout has been pushing back against the sexualisation of breast cancer awareness, urging companies to focus on saving people, not breasts. They highlight a number of examples from recent years, from hypersexualised 'breast check' posters, to food shaped as disembodied breasts, to a company changing their name to 'Boobs' for the month of October.[40] While I do not agree with all of the viewpoints of this group, particularly their stance around sex work,

I do believe there is a time and a place for sexualisation and that place is not in raising awareness for a deadly disease – particularly in a way that is both figuratively and literally removed from the faces and lives of the people who are affected.

I have struggled with where to focus my advocacy because even the organisations that are doing good work often partner with these companies who engage in sexualisation, accepting the small percentage of the profits that is offered up in exchange for the legitimacy of the charity's name across their website and social media. I understand that the work of raising money for charity is hard and these partnerships are often entered into with the best of intentions, but having been through the horrible secret shroud and into the world of a cancer patient, I don't feel like I can be involved with causes that glamorise and sexualise something so acutely awful.

While writing Sophie's story, I was so impressed with the work of Professor Caroline Ford. Professor Ford started out in breast cancer research, but moved into ovarian cancer and other gynaecological cancers when she discovered how severely under-researched they are. The partnership she has forged with Camilla and Marc has been really purposeful and meaningful – while it likely also helps drive profits for the brand, something that is almost unavoidable under capitalism, it remains connected to people whose lives have been affected by ovarian cancer and it has a specific aim in raising money for an early detection test.

And so slowly, subconsciously, I have been allowing my thoughts to twist around the idea of different types of advocacy for different causes. It is not as straightforward as simply being an advocate in the breast cancer space would be. It means less reliance on my lived experience and making sure not to speak over the voices of people who have been deeply affected by the diseases and traumas. But the idea of advocating through fundraising and amplification of the voices of survivors and family members calls to me more and more often.

Through the stories of these young advocates, I have come to understand that advocacy can bring healing, but it needs to be the right cause and the right time. All three described the feelings of powerlessness that plagued them during their own or their loved ones' illnesses and the way being able to do something and make a difference for the people who came after helped them step into their own power. Amy described it as feeling like the hole in her heart, created by her mother's illness, started to get smaller when she was able to contribute in some way. I have not yet found exactly what it is that will help the hole in my own heart start to get smaller. But through these discussions and thinking more deeply and laterally about the possibilities of advocacy, I feel like I am at least on the path to finding it.

CHAPTER SEVEN

Linger

'Feeling lucky makes you less likely to focus on bad things in your life.'

Walking home from the train station after work one day, I hurried to overtake some slow walkers. I have no patience for slow walkers – even my own experience of being sick and living life at a slower pace has not helped in this regard. This particular group was taking up the entire path and I had to veer onto the nature strip beside the road to get around them. As I did, my foot caught on the join between the footpath and grass and my ankle rolled slightly. It's not an unusual thing to happen to me, but where previously I would have just steadied myself and continued walking, this time, something felt different.

I couldn't get my balance and I hit the ground hard. The group of slow walkers turned to look at me. I was okay – just grazed knees and wounded pride – but I couldn't understand why I ended up on the ground. I decided it must have been age-related – at thirty-eight, maybe I was entering the period of my life where people no longer say that I fell over, but instead that I 'had a fall'. I didn't think too much more about it.

Months later, I was at the gym, with a new trainer leading the class. The trainer happened to be a friend of mine, but I hadn't done a class with her before. At the end of the strength class, she gave us balance exercises to finish. I stepped into them confidently – I did gymnastics as a kid and have always had good balance – but the simple exercise immediately gave me problems. My ankles wobbled with instability. I was constantly bringing my foot down, starting again. I couldn't seem to get my body to work in the way that it used to. Later that night, I remembered my fall on the street. The cogs in my brain began turning and remembered something I had heard others mention in cancer forums. I pulled up Google on my phone and typed 'chemo balance problems'. The list of results was long and included numerous peer-reviewed studies investigating the relationship between chemotherapy and ongoing issues with balance.

Over the next few months, things got worse. I rolled my ankle badly twice – once jumping down from a small ledge onto the grass at the zoo and the other time simply walking along the street. In between, I had other smaller falls. I no longer felt safe even glancing down at my phone while walking. I needed to give all my attention to putting one foot in front of the other. This experience was the closest I've come to melting down in my post-cancer era. I felt furious that my body had betrayed me. I have never been a natural athlete, but I have always been fitter and more able than the average person. The inability to do something as simple as walk without fear of falling was simply unthinkable. The lack of control I felt was upsetting, but what was even worse was the fact that I thought all this was behind me. I did the hard part – I made it through surgery, chemo and radiation. Life should be going back to normal, not throwing me endless new curveballs.

After sitting with this feeling for a few weeks, caught between despair and anger, I decided to bring it up with my oncologist at my next appointment. The day arrived and when I finished explaining, she considered the question. 'It's been over a year since you finished chemotherapy,' she reminded me. 'Have you got much peripheral neuropathy still?'

Peripheral neuropathy is a side effect from chemo that results in numbness to the hands and feet. I was lucky not to experience too much of this particular side effect, as it can be incredibly disruptive to people's lives.

'Only in the tips of my thumbs,' I told her.

'In that case, I don't think it's related,' she said. 'People have balance issues from chemotherapy because they can't feel their toes and feet properly, but you don't have that issue. I understand that when you've had cancer there's a tendency to want to attribute everything you experience to that, but some things are just not because of cancer.'

From that time on, I tried to forget about it and just focus on not falling over so much. I started wearing thick rubber boots that come up over my ankles everywhere I went because they provided the stability to stop me from falling most of the time. I resisted the temptation to check messages that came through while walking, because any distraction could send me toppling over. Even now, every time I walk, all I am focused on is the next step I take and staying on my feet. It is frustrating, but it mostly works in stopping the falls. But the lingering feeling has remained that I went from being someone who had good balance to someone who had terrible balance and cancer treatment was the only thing in between. And so, I went back to investigating and found new research – specifically in breast cancer patients who have had chemotherapy – that suggests a high level of fatigue during, and persisting after, chemo may be a bigger factor than peripheral neuropathy in the development of long-term balance issues. The results of the study indicate that 'cancer-related fatigue, even several years following exposure to chemotherapy, may distinctly influence balance independent of a patient's chemotherapy-induced peripheral neuropathy status.'[41]

Fatigue is certainly the side effect I felt most acutely during chemo and the effects have persisted long after. While it is nothing compared to those days I spent in bed, unable to do anything, I know I have to be careful with what I commit to in my post-cancer life, that simply living life at the same pace I did before can knock me around for days and leave me feeling exhausted and unwell. These lingering physical side effects are annoying at their best and incredibly disruptive at their worst. While I don't always know if I can attribute these difficulties to chemo or cancer, I do know that I feel like a physically different person to who I was before. I am nowhere near as fit, my body has changed shape and my hair has grown back differently; I find it hard to be the person I was before cancer when I feel so far removed from that person on even a basic, physical level.

The ongoing mental and emotional side effects show no sign of dissipating either. They show themselves in sometimes peculiar ways. Every so often, I'll be in the middle of some mundane frustration when I remember that I should be grateful. Recently, I was heading out to pick my daughter up from an art class and my phone wouldn't connect to the car. I tried multiple times, but it just wouldn't happen. Consequently, I missed the turn-off because I decided I'd be fine to rely on my memory rather than Google Maps, and ended up lost and stuck in traffic, panicked about being late. In the midst of losing my shit about all this, I had the sudden thought, *Yes, but at least you're alive!*

My subconscious decided that was the right moment to become heavily into toxic positivity and it was that more than any of the previous frustrations that nearly pushed me over the edge. In her *New York Times* essay 'My Transplanted Heart and I Will Die Soon', Amy Silverstein describes this as the 'gratitude paradox'.

'Because a transplant begins with the overwhelming gift of a donor organ that brings you back from the brink of death, the entirety of a patient's experience from that day forward is cast as a "miracle",' she writes. 'And who doesn't love a good miracle story? But this narrative discourages transplant recipients from talking freely about the real problems we face and the compromising and life-threatening side effects of the medicines we must take.'[42]

Silverstein speaks about the vitriol she received after writing about her full range of emotions following her heart transplant. While I have not experienced that level of public scrutiny or external insistence on gratitude, I have internalised this idea that living after a potentially fatal illness requires me to be grateful for every moment. That I am no longer entitled to frustrations that plague regular people. I must rise above these, floating on the pure bliss of the years of life I stole back. No doubt there is a gendered element to this feeling – gratitude often seems to be compulsory for women and other marginalised people. Even during the Women's Marches in 2021, which protested against gendered violence, then Prime Minister Scott Morrison tried to invoke gratitude from the protestors for the fact that they were not met with violence while marching.

'Not far from here, such marches, even now are being met with bullets, but not here in this country,' he said in Parliament. 'This is a triumph of democracy when we see these things take place.'

This internalised focus on gratitude was something I did not fully consider when I imagined life after cancer treatment. I pictured a tough year of sickness and side effects, which may take a little while to recover from, but by now I had expected it would be behind me, just a story to tell about something that had once happened to me. I didn't expect to be this tired, slow, constantly falling over person who can't quite manage to be as grateful as she thinks she should be, who still feels emotionally stunted and not as mentally switched on as she once was. I underestimated the ways the ongoing effects of my trauma would impact me and I'm struggling now to allow space for them without giving them too much focus.

In order to better understand how to do that, I decide to speak to someone who has carved out a life after trauma over many years and has found peace amid its lingering influence.

AJ

I have known AJ for a long time, although we have only met in person a handful of times. She lives far from me, in a small regional town, and we have caught up a few times when she has visited Sydney for work, or when we have both been in Melbourne. We met through an online forum and have maintained a friendship over social media. AJ is an unfailingly kind and lovely person – she sent gifts to Pia during lockdown, completely unprompted, because she knew it must be tough to be a child stuck at home, unable to see any friends. When I asked on Twitter for suggestions about where to buy scarves when my hair was falling out during chemo, rather than make a suggestion, she ordered a few beautiful scarves online and had them sent to me. She is fairly universally beloved in our social media circles, which is an extremely rare thing in any online space. She is, in short, a very special person.

AJ's trauma stretches back many years, to when she was sexually abused by a priest at just five years old. Although it took her years to fully understand everything that had happened to her, the trauma was ever-present throughout her childhood, weaving its way into every aspect of her life. We speak about it one afternoon, the sun creeping in through my window and AJ's gentle but confident voice washing over me.

'One of the periods when I started to properly understand what had happened was when I was about eleven, and starting to go through puberty, learning about sex and things like that,' she says. 'I still didn't fully understand it, but I became very, very angry. Just knowing that it had happened, and that it shouldn't have. But I couldn't really articulate it, even to myself.'

As the understanding grew, it seemed to take up more space inside AJ than she could cope with, and the trauma began to escape in ways that she couldn't explain to her family. She felt constantly on edge, which often tipped into anger that took over her body. 'I remember that I used to go into these rages sometimes,' she says. 'I was so angry, and it really affected my parents and sisters especially. My older brother had left home by the time this started, so it didn't affect him as much. But I had one sister three years older, and one a year younger, and they couldn't understand why I was like that. I couldn't understand it myself.'

AJ's rage seemed to leap out of her at unexpected times and assert itself in increasingly uncontrolled ways. 'I tore up a lot of photos, and back then photos were very expensive,' she says. 'We didn't have many photos of us as kids and I ripped up a lot of them – especially any I found of me as a child. Then when I was about fifteen, I started drinking heavily, getting into a lot of risky behaviour in my later teens and sleeping with random people.'

AJ carried her trauma with her for many years before she began to process it. Even once she started to understand it better and felt able to explain it, she continued to carry a lot of guilt, shame and fear that no-one would believe her. Eventually, a culmination of an increasing number of media stories about child sexual abuse spurred her to action. 'I started to get this increasing feeling that I was going to one day explode inappropriately about what had happened,' she says. 'I realised I needed to address it because I didn't want to be at work and start disclosing when it wasn't the right time for me. So I started to think about it more and more. I drive a lot for work, so I had a lot of time to think.'

Through her work, AJ was aware of Knowmore – a free, independent legal service for survivors of child sexual abuse – and after many hours of thinking about it on the road, she summoned the courage to report the abuse she had suffered. 'That first phone call was pretty amazing, in the scheme of things,' she says. 'I rang up and spoke to an intake worker who told me I probably wouldn't get an appointment for about eight weeks, but they wanted to make sure I was okay. The person said, "I'm really sorry this happened to you and I want to tell you that we believe you." I think just having someone say those words, I broke down – it was like this massive pressure valve had gone off.'

Over the next weeks and months, AJ spoke with the staff at Knowmore a few more times, always finding them incredibly kind and understanding. There was a long wait for an appointment, but through her phone conversations, she began to feel confident and empowered enough to begin an application to the National Redress Scheme on her own.

The National Redress Scheme was set up in response to the Australian Royal Commission into Institutional

Responses to Child Sexual Abuse. It was designed to give people who experienced institutional child sexual abuse access to counselling, a direct personal response from the institution responsible for the abuse – which can include an apology and the steps being taken to prevent it from happening in the future – and a redress payment. It took AJ almost a month to complete the application, due to the emotions it brought up for her.

'It was pretty harrowing,' she says. 'At that stage, I had told nobody – I hadn't told my husband, I hadn't told anybody at all in my life. So it was quite difficult. I kept putting it aside and going back to it when I felt up to it. I also didn't want to rush it because as time went on, and I started thinking more about it, I started to understand a lot of the effects that it had on me and I was able to add more detail.'

Once she had lodged the application, it took a year before she received the outcome. It was a stressful time. The delay was due to caseworkers leaving and her application falling through the cracks of the system on a number of occasions. Once the information had been verified, it was reviewed by an independent panel and scored on a matrix to determine the outcome and payout.

'Every person I dealt with was amazing, even though it was a bit frustrating at times with the delays,' she says.

'Everyone was very kind, they apologised that I had to go through this, they told me that they understood that it was a distressing process. They obviously got the right people and that was a good thing, because I think for so many people like myself to actually take that step to do something about it, if the people you had to deal with were rude or dismissive, then it just would have made the whole process so much worse.'

AJ finally received her response and a payout. She expected to feel relieved and joyful once the outcome was decided, but the reality was more complex. 'I felt really mixed, actually ... Before I got it, I had thought I wanted to buy myself something really significant, but I didn't know what, so I put that money aside,' she says. 'I used some of it to buy a car, but I still haven't bought anything personal with it. I think the longer time went on, the less I needed to.'

The part of the compensation that AJ found the most useful was the access to counselling sessions. She was provided with a list of counsellors in her area that she could speak to and received twenty free sessions. 'The counselling has been a huge part of me being able to move on and I was really lucky that I got someone who I clicked with straight away,' she says. 'Initially, I probably went every couple of weeks, but sometimes now I've had four months between going and then something will come up and I think, oh, gosh, I need to go and talk to her.'

The most immediate thing her counsellor was able to help with was how to cope when triggers came up. AJ found that these were often connected with child sexual abuse stories in the media. 'George Pell's death was a huge trigger for me,' she says. 'Even though he wasn't involved in my situation, for me, he has been a symbol of the Church covering things up. Some of the publicity from people speaking out and saying that he was a saint and he never did anything wrong was difficult to hear as well. So having my counsellor to talk to and help me understand what I'm feeling and how to deal with those feelings has been so important.'

AJ's counsellor also helped her make a plan to be able to talk to key people in her life about what happened to her. She had told her husband once she submitted the claim, but she wanted some support to help her tell her daughter and sisters. This was more confronting than disclosing to the strangers on the phone. 'It was really important for me to tell my sisters, but I had to be in the right headspace to do it,' she says. 'My counsellor worked a lot with me to be able to tell them. We worked on it for longer than I had expected because of bloody Covid! I wanted to tell them in person and they're both in Adelaide. I was really prepared to tell them on a couple of occasions and then I couldn't go and so that was really stressful.'

AJ knew her sisters would be devastated when they found out what had happened to her, but she wasn't in a position to take on their devastation. So she worked hard on getting the wording right and running through all the possible scenarios of how the conversation might go with her counsellor so she would be prepared to say the right things. Eventually, she got her opportunity to travel to Adelaide and see them. 'I was staying with one sister and I asked my other sister if she was doing anything that afternoon,' she says. 'I suggested a walk on the beach. I didn't want to make a big deal of telling them I had to talk to them about something, because I didn't want them worrying or trying to figure out what it could be. But the whole time we were walking, I just kept thinking, oh, god, I've got to do it, I have to do it now.'

AJ asked her sisters to sit down and told them the news she had been holding inside her for so long. Although it was hard for them to hear, she was glad that the moment had finally come and she was able to release a bit more of the pressure that had been building up. 'It was a huge relief for me to be able to tell them,' she says. 'Obviously they were really upset and angry, but by that stage, I was in a pretty good place with it.'

The long wait to tell her sisters was helpful in the end, because AJ felt confident in her ability to reassure them without taking their hurt and pain on herself. 'By waiting to tell them, I felt comfortable saying, "I know this is really hard for you to hear, because this is so new for you, but it's not for me",' she says. 'That was some of the language that my counsellor helped me with. I told them that I was okay and I was at the stage where I was dealing with it and I needed to tell people who were important to me.'

Having this conversation was particularly significant to AJ because she wanted her sisters to understand her behaviour as a child and a teenager. They had been with her while she wrestled with this inner turmoil, but it wasn't until this moment that they were able to fully grasp it. 'It explained so much, particularly for my younger sister, because we were only a year apart,' she says. 'We've had conversations since where she's said, "I'm so glad you told me because I always thought something was wrong with me and that's why you were always so angry with me." It's upsetting to hear of the effect on somebody else. But even though we've always been pretty close as adults, telling them has definitely made a difference in our relationship; they now really get why I was the way I was.'

The other important conversation AJ needed to have was with her daughter. By this stage, her daughter had grown up, was living out of home with her husband and was pregnant. Fortunately, she still lived close by and AJ did not have the long Covid delays in being able to talk to her about it. 'I was really glad that I told her,' she says. 'She's a really mature young person. She was upset about it, but she took it well and had a really good response to it. My counsellor helped me prepare for that conversation as well, because I knew it would be upsetting for her and I wanted to get it right.'

AJ wanted to make sure her daughter understood what had happened in part because she felt the echoes of her trauma had left their mark on her parenting and – like with her sisters – she felt it would help make sense of some of her behaviour. 'I was always very cautious as a parent,' she says. 'I did send her to a Catholic school, but being in a regional area, there's often not a lot of choice. But I found it hard sometimes when she would ask me to come to something they had on at school and it was in the church, because I really didn't like going into churches.'

AJ also found it difficult when her daughter was invited to sleepovers, with the memory of what had happened to her at such a young age ever-present in her mind. 'She did have sleepovers, but they were with, as far as you can ever know, people that I trusted,' she says. 'Then as she was getting older, I was really conscious of making sure she knew that she could tell me anything. Even at that time, conversations around consent weren't such a big thing, but I was probably a lot more vigilant around safety and who she was spending time with than I perhaps might have been otherwise.'

While the discussions she had with her daughter and sisters were therapeutic and important, AJ made a conscious decision at the start of the process not to inform her parents. At the time she was starting down the path of reporting her experience, they were in their eighties and she did not feel it would be helpful for them to know.

'There was just going to be no good that would come from telling them,' she says of her parents, who have since died. 'Even though it might have explained a lot from when I was a teenager. But that was such a long time ago, I didn't think it was as important for them as it was for my sisters. I knew that it would have been extremely upsetting for them. So I didn't ever think that I would tell them.'

AJ also has her doubts about what they would have said to her if she had told them, particularly if she had done so when she was younger. 'They were very devout Catholics,' she says. 'I don't really know whether they would have even believed me had I told them when I was younger. There was always the belief that priests and nuns can do no wrong, like there was for a lot of people of that era.'

AJ is working in a job that she loves, which involves running education sessions for young people about consent. While she initially had some concerns about how she would cope, she has found it surprisingly straightforward.

'I've probably done a couple of hundred of those sessions now,' she says. 'I don't find it triggering at all. I find it a bit cathartic, I suppose. It's really important to me that young people get this education – even having mandatory consent education from primary school, not necessarily around sexual consent, but learning what consent is, will make it easier for young people to make those disclosures and know that perhaps something isn't right. The sessions have been a really good thing that we've been doing, and I think they've been good for me too.'

The feeling of making a difference, of doing something to help, brings to mind Amy, Molly and Sophie's experiences and my own desire to find healing through advocacy. AJ feels that advocacy is in her future, but for now she is not quite ready to embark on that journey and what she is doing through her work is enough. 'I do want to be a bit more down the track in processing it all,' she says. 'At the moment, I can still be intensely triggered at times. I don't think those triggers will ever fully go away, but I know I'm not ready just yet.'

Until that day comes, AJ feels at peace with the person she has become and the way she has processed her trauma. Interestingly, one of the most important factors for her has been sitting with a sense of gratitude for the life she has built. It is something she has incorporated into her life for a long time. 'I always wanted a big family and I only ended up with one child for various reasons,' she says. 'I had a realisation one day when I was really sad after having a couple of miscarriages. I thought, if it's not going to happen, do I want to be miserable and not appreciate her? I've got one perfect child, I need to do the best I can to be happy about that. I think that was a big realisation for me; if I've only got one, I really want to bloody enjoy her!'

AJ has carried that gratitude for her child through her life and finds it has helped her through some dark times. 'I always say to her, "I feel blessed every day that I'm your mum." She's brought me so much joy. She's a pretty awesome young woman, and I just feel so proud of her. It makes me think that I did do something right, even though I was going through all this.'

She also finds gratitude in the time she spends with her granddaughter, who is the light of her life. Her granddaughter was born just months after AJ's mother died and she has found her presence to be healing. 'My daughter said when she found out that she was pregnant, "I just feel like this is a turning of the page, and it's going to be a good thing that's happened to our family,"' AJ remembers. 'It certainly was because my granddaughter brings me so much joy. I have her with me every Friday and I just love that time with her. She's a real little character.'

Spending time with her granddaughter has also pushed her to live in the moment and focus on the joy that is right in front of her. 'I think feeling so lucky makes you less likely to focus on bad things in your life,' she says. 'How can I wallow in something that's happened to me – even though it was very traumatising – when I have her in my life?'

As the years have gone by, AJ has begun to feel more comfortable with herself. She is now at a point where she has processed the trauma and does not allow it to take up as much space in her life. Although her life is one that will always be marked by trauma, she is no longer defined by it. Through her own hard work, incredible spirit and the love of those around her, she redefined her life as something truly special. When she thinks back on her younger self, her memories are tinged with sadness, but ultimately, she sees hope and recovery.

'If I could go back and talk to that little girl, I would say, "You're going to have a good life. It might not seem like it now, but things will be okay,' she says. 'I know that I'm really lucky that I have been able to build a life where, while it has affected me, I've also been married nearly thirty years, I've got really good relationships with my family. I don't have any substance abuse problems. I'm in a job that I love. Those are all things that a lot of people in my position don't have, so I do count myself extremely lucky. So I'd just want that little girl to know that it is going to be okay.'

It's a beautiful message and one that will continue to guide her forward. Though she should never have had to endure the pain, the life she has created from its wreckage is a special one and well worth living.

* * *

What remains in my mind long after my chat with AJ is the way she expresses her gratitude. While I had previously considered gratitude as something that requires falling into the traps of toxic positivity, something from the realms of dreamy inspirational quotes that are reposted on Instagram ad nauseam, AJ has shown me that gratitude can be more humble and genuine. She does not allow it to nullify her trauma or admonish herself for continuing to find it hard to live with her experience of child sexual abuse. Instead of pulling her gratitude down over the top of her trauma and trying to completely block it out, she allows the two states of being to sit side-by-side. The light of her gratitude leaks gently into the darkness of her trauma, but she does not insist that it becomes bright enough to blast the shadows away. She is content to sit with both experiences.

This nudges me into considering what I am grateful for in my own life, though I have fought doing that before now, feeling grumpy at the idea that I *have* to appreciate things. Above all, my gratitude is for my life itself. I feel now that I can be grateful that I am alive while still feeling sad about what I lost and allowing myself to get annoyed about inconveniences. Having been confronted with death – with the idea of not seeing my daughter grow up – I now see the fragility of life and understand that this fragility is part of what makes it so beautiful. Once I start thinking about this, I can't stop, the thoughts tumbling down as if they had been poised on a precipice, waiting for me to be ready to let them in.

I am grateful for Pia, for the pure love she exudes, the incredible energy she possesses, the passion, loyalty and utter silliness that make her up.

I am grateful for Shaun, the person who makes me laugh more than anyone else in the world, who loves Pia and me unendingly and who did absolutely everything I could have hoped for and more while I was sick, without me needing to ask.

For my mum, who is the strongest person I know and who threw her whole self into helping me while I was sick, from being my font of medical knowledge to babysitting and everything in between. Who told me that she wished she could have taken the cancer from me and endured it instead, so upsetting was it for her to see me suffer through it.

For my dad, who called me when a friend told him that cancer treatment can be expensive and told me never to worry about money, that he would always take care of me.

For my friends who came and sat with me, or brought me food or sent me gifts – and even for the ones who didn't know what to do and wanted me to tell them what I needed. I'm so grateful that they cared enough to ask.

Now that I have started letting this gratitude in, I feel like I could go on forever. I have spent so long resenting the idea of gratitude that it feels almost revolutionary to let it wash over me. The way AJ spoke about her daughter and granddaughter was so joyful and gracious and it feels like it has opened a floodgate in me. It has given me a new way to think about the lingering side effects of illness, treatment and trauma. I can let them – and my feelings about them – sit side-by-side with moments of gratitude and joy. I had been thinking of these states as mutually exclusive – that I needed to process or even eliminate the negativity I feel before I had time for other feelings. Or that expressing gratitude somehow lessens what I have been through. It sounds ridiculously simple – I struggle to write it down because I can imagine everyone reading it throwing the book away and rolling their eyes about what an obvious conclusion I have drawn. Why did I need to dig into all these other stories just to realise that I could have negative and positive feelings at once? But my clouded brain was not ready to understand this until now and I realise that others who have experienced trauma may feel the same way, so it feels important to articulate.

In her article published in *The Guardian*, 'Is gratitude the secret of happiness?', Moya Sarner writes about grappling with some of those same feelings about the concept of gratitude that I struggled with. 'The notion of formalised, prescribed and premeditated gratitude, which in the past decade has become the darling of positive psychology and the self-help movement, tends to stick in my craw,' she writes. 'I am too cynical to get on board this particular Oprah bandwagon – too British, too atheist, too sensitive to schmaltz.'[43]

However, Sarner discovers that the science is there to support the link between gratitude and wellbeing, linking it to everything from decreased levels of anxiety and depression to better sleep and body image. Like me, once she began to take the time to think about what she is grateful for, the floodgates opened and she felt 'a warm, settled, comforting feeling' as the process of keeping a gratitude journal began to form part of her day.

A 2017 study conducted by the University of Sheffield and the University of Stirling specifically looked at gratitude in relation to people with chronic illness, which interested me. It is one thing to be grateful when life is easy, but what effect could gratitude have on people for whom life is a struggle, people who may not feel they have much to be grateful for? The researchers found that higher levels of gratitude were closely associated with lower levels of depressive symptoms, even when other differentiating factors were controlled for.[44] Another study by Brock University in 2011 looked at gratitude in people with traumatic spinal cord injuries. This study also found that when participants were able to view the extreme challenges in their lives through a lens of positivity and gratitude, with the help of guided interventions, their wellbeing improved.[45]

These studies are interesting and I'm glad I read them after speaking with AJ. I needed to reframe the idea of gratitude and the unique space it can take up in order to move away from resenting the entire concept. I now understand the way the threads of gratitude can join together with the lingering effects of trauma to weave a more complex pattern into a life.

While I know that simply being grateful is not the answer to all the problems of the world, I now feel better equipped to let it in and make it part of the way I go on in the world. I am grateful for my life, and that does not mean ignoring its difficulties. For now, at least, I must be content to sit with more complex feelings.

CHAPTER EIGHT

Leaps and Bounds

As I pull on my purple and yellow netball uniform, the feeling is a little surreal. It has been 687 days since I last stepped on to a netball court. In comparison to some of my teammates, who are returning to netball in their fifties having last played in high school, it is nothing. But for me, this is a moment, maybe even *the* moment, in my recovery. I first started playing netball in 1992 and this is the longest break I have ever had from playing the sport I fell in love with as a seven-year-old. The only other significant break was when I was pregnant with Pia.

The afternoon is rain-soaked and chilly. The asphalt courts are slick with water and there are few people around to witness this. I remember interviewing former Australian netball captain Liz Ellis about the game when she made her return from an anterior cruciate ligament injury. It was a state league game, held in Sydney's western suburbs, with barely a spectator in sight. It seemed far removed from the game where she had sustained her injury – a fiercely fought battle against New Zealand in front of thousands of screaming fans. In comparison, her return felt small and lonely. But to her, it was everything.

My own return is even smaller. Shaun and Pia have come to see me play, but the rest of the sideline is as deserted as you would expect a C-grade netball game to be on a drizzly Saturday afternoon. As a result, I feel almost dissociated from what is happening. What I have been through to get back here has been so huge that in my mind I feel I should have a stadium full of people cheering as it happens. Of course, they would probably be a disappointed stadium once they saw me slowly loping around the court after the ball, but in my mind's eye, they are all very supportive.

In my time away from playing, one thing has not changed. No-one wants to play centre – the position that requires the most running – so despite my tired body that feels much older than its thirty-eight years, I take the C bib and press the velcro squares to my shirt. I take the ball and walk to the centre circle to begin the game.

* * *

It took some time for me to be ready to play netball. My final chemo session was in late April 2022, only a few weeks into the netball season, so originally I thought I might just miss the first few weeks and then jump straight back into playing. I greatly underestimated the ongoing effects of pumping poison into my body on a weekly basis for six months. While I soon realised that netball would have to wait a little longer, I sought the comfort of exercise and moving my body. It is something I have always done and life didn't feel quite right without it.

My friend Ana had recently started going to a gym in the next suburb. I have dipped in and out of gyms over the years – I enjoy group exercise classes but often find the style of teaching to be about pushing yourself to an uncomfortable point, and I was not able to cope with being unable to meet the expectations. I had also got to a point where I was thinking differently about my body. For most of my life, I was a thin person and I judged myself harshly every time I let my body slip away from that standard. Even when I was very thin – wearing size six clothing – I hated that my stomach was not completely flat and I severely restricted my calories to try to achieve this 'ideal' body. But after pregnancy and childbirth, the shape of my body changed. I still wore straight sized clothes, but I didn't feel like I was in the body I should be in. Cancer treatment again played havoc with my body shape and image – steroids caused my face to puff up during treatment, I lost my hair, eyebrows and eyelashes and chemical menopause messed with my metabolism. I was still by no means in the kind of body that is stigmatised and discriminated against, but neither was I comfortable in a gym setting where the focus is on achieving and maintaining a very thin and muscular body.

The gym that Ana had signed up for sounded different. I had a look at their website and found a description that seemed like exactly what I was looking for. 'Haven is a special body-affirming space designed to help our members cultivate a peaceful relationship with their bodies through movement, yoga and self-compassion. We're proudly fat-positive, non-diet and weight-inclusive – meaning we don't focus on weight loss, rather we neutralise body size and gently draw your attention to enjoying movement and caring for your body – not controlling it, shrinking it or judging it.'[46]

After years of judging my own body and trying desperately to shrink it, I was bigger than I had ever been before and all I wanted was to be able to accept it. The gym's owner, Anna, meets every potential client for a cup of tea and discussion of their needs before they sign up, to make sure they understand the values of the gym and so she learns what she can do to support their goals. During our meeting, I found out that the gym had exercise physiologists and that my cancer qualified me to have some sessions subsidised by Medicare. I was still completing chemo when I first started to see my exercise physiologist. Ellen was like a human ray of sunshine. Every session, she seemed to have a new hair colour and different fun and quirky earrings. We started slowly and she taught me how to exercise without pushing myself to the limits of my comfort zone. I learned that it was okay to be gentle with my body, to move it slowly, and that there was no need to feel guilty if I walked away from a session not dripping with sweat and feeling like vomiting. In fact, in my current condition, it was greatly preferred.

It was a radical way for me to think about exercise. Prior to my pregnancy, I had been extremely into running and there were days when I only felt like I could manage four or five kilometres. But so warped was my perception of what exercise should be that many times I opted to do nothing at all, because anything less than ten kilometres felt like a waste. The idea of exercising without pushing myself to the limit was a concept I simply had not entertained before.

With Ellen, I learned to be kind to myself and to listen to my body. It was something I had struggled with throughout chemo, as I convinced myself of my ability to push through the pain, nausea and fatigue and try to live as normal a life as possible. Ellen's trauma-informed approach to exercise, which involved elements of motivational interviewing, cognitive behavioural therapy and acceptance and commitment therapy, helped me to find the joy in movement again and not think of exercise as a punishment for eating the 'wrong' foods.

Over the months, I began to regain my strength and try new things. I had never been particularly interested in weight training, as I wasn't naturally good at it and like many women who were once bright girls, I had a belief that anything that didn't come naturally to me was something I was unable to conquer. But in the absence of my ability to do cardio exercises to my usual standard – and because I had been reading studies about the link between weight training and reducing breast cancer recurrence risk – I dived in headfirst and let Ellen teach me how to lift.

It took time to do it without judgement. Often I would be working with Ellen at the same time other people in the gym were doing personal training sessions. They all seemed so much stronger than me, lifting heavy weights with ease, while I started with just the empty – but decidedly heavy – bar. I always felt like I should be doing more, should be better at it, but gradually, I learned to quiet that impulse and focus on myself. I got stronger and more able, finding ways to quietly challenge myself without feeling like I needed to be constantly pushed to my limit. The more I exercised, the better I felt.

As the weeks and months of my recovery went on, even as I found myself stronger and more confident, I couldn't shake the feeling that I was new to all this. After regaining my strength and confidence with Ellen, I started to move back into the spaces I had once occupied and found them unfamiliar.

It was a strange feeling for someone whose whole life has been so connected with sport. I returned to sport so I could find my way back to the person I was before. On the netball court and the running track, I had always felt like myself and I expected that feeling to be there, waiting for me, when I returned.

When I didn't find it in that first netball game, when the person who put on the centre bib was slower and less adept than the person I had left behind on that court 687 days earlier, I tried not to let it worry me. I thought I might find more of myself throughout that season, that little by little I would return to being myself, simply through the magic of passing a ball around an asphalt court for sixty minutes every Saturday afternoon. But the more weeks went by, the less sure I felt. Each game left me feeling empty and alone; the person I was looking for wasn't there.

It has taken me a long time to come to terms with that loss – or even to articulate it. Throughout my illness, I had idolised New Zealand football player Rebekah Stott, who had returned to play at the highest level after recovering from Hodgkin's lymphoma, and Colombian footballer Linda Caicedo, who lit up the World Cup three years after being diagnosed with ovarian cancer. While I am well aware that I am nowhere near the level of an elite athlete, that they seemed to step so seamlessly into their old selves gave me hope that I could do the same. I held no delusions about playing in a World Cup, but I did think I could find a way to pick up where I left off. Instead, I felt like a stranger in my own body and mind, muddling through something that used to come easily.

I thought maybe running was a better place to start – with just me and the path, surely it would be harder to go wrong? Pia wanted to train for her school cross-country race, so I embarked on a two-kilometre run with her. In my former life, two kilometres would barely have registered as a run for me, so I thought it would be no problem while still completing chemo. I made it through the distance, but just barely. As soon as we finished, I sank to the ground and struggled to regain my breath and my sense of the world. The pace was slower than anything I had ever run, but it was so hard. I felt like I was running through waist-deep mud. Over time, it has slowly become easier, but the differences have felt incremental.

Over a year after completing treatment, I ran in my first post-cancer fun run. It was a five-kilometre event and out of habit, I picked my way through the crowd and positioned myself where I would usually start from – close to but not right at the front. I overheard some runners near me talk about their aim to complete the course in twenty-three minutes. I absentmindedly edged closer, thinking for a second that I was in the right place, that I could follow these people who were planning to run the race in my personal best time for five kilometres. By the time I remembered that I would be lucky to come within ten minutes of that time, we were off and I had to move myself over to the left and make sure I was out of the way of all these much faster runners leaving me in their wake.

I ran the full distance – nowhere near that personal best time, of course – but I made it to the end. The whole time I was running, all those thousands of steps I took, all I could think about was how hard it was. I never felt like I was able to get into a rhythm or let momentum carry me through for even a couple of steps. I couldn't understand how I felt so fundamentally changed after a relatively short break from running. My muscle memory had been completely erased and after more than a year, I had not made much progress in rebuilding it. It felt like I was starting from scratch in a new body, one that had no connection to who I was before. I thought that I could find myself again in sport, but instead, I felt even more lost. I wanted to understand more about the relationship between exercise and trauma, to find some knowledge that would help me process the strange, empty feelings I was having.

In her book *Lifting Heavy Things: Healing Trauma One Rep at a Time*, Laura Khoudari explores the relationship between exercise and recovery from trauma. Khoudari became a personal trainer – with a particular focus on strength training – after recovery from a trauma in her past, which she never details in her book, only marking the space with [ ] whenever it comes up. Khoudari grew tired of the 'exclusionary' culture in traditional gyms and sought out spaces where people of all sizes were included and celebrated. Her book switched on a lot of lightbulbs in my mind as I read about her experiences helping people heal their minds and bodies at the same time.

'Recovery doesn't look like just going back to "normal" for any of your parts: when your muscles recover from strength training they don't just feel better, they physically change and get stronger,' she writes. 'The same can be said about recovering from trauma. The fact is that the trauma happened. If you can integrate it into your story instead of having it dominate your narrative, including your relationships, you will make space to recover—not just to feel better, but stronger.'[47]

The more I read and speak to people, the more I discover others who have found healing from trauma in exercise. From professional athletes returning to play sport at the highest level to everyday people who started taking themselves for walks to pass the time and found joy in movement, there is plenty of evidence to suggest that exercise can be beneficial for people who have suffered all different kinds of trauma. Studies have found that incorporating exercise into a recovery program for people with PTSD can help to reduce their symptoms.[48] Recently, work has been done in creating specific exercise programs for survivors of trauma to meet their specific needs in their recovery – for instance, programs for female survivors of sexual violence have been most effective when they are available to women in their homes and offer female instructors.[49]

The idea of exercise as a specific healing tool is an interesting one, but it is not without complexities.

People with mental illness are often advised to exercise as a way to improve their mental health, but this advice can be fraught. Most people don't dispute that exercise is indeed incredibly beneficial, but for people who are in the middle of a major depressive episode, or are dealing with the more complex symptoms of illnesses like bipolar or schizophrenia, it is not as easy as just deciding to get up and go for a run or join a soccer team. Similarly, for people who are living with other chronic illnesses, who need to manage pain and fatigue on a daily basis, sometimes exercise simply isn't an option, no matter how gentle. I think that's the most frustrating thing about it – everyone knows it helps, but sometimes it isn't possible.

Scrolling through Instagram one day, I see a video posted by a breast cancer surgeon who is also a breast cancer patient. In the video, she is sweaty after a run, talking to the camera and telling the breast cancer patients who follow her to get off the couch, as it's the best thing for dealing with fatigue. It goes down as well as you would expect. People are upset and anxious about something that feels akin to a guilt trip while they're going through the most difficult time of their lives. The surgeon did not mean to strike a nerve or upset anyone, but it was something I could see coming from a mile away, as someone who has been immersed in the sensitivities and vulnerabilities around exercise.

The relationship between women and physical activity is a long and complicated one. Women have traditionally been locked out of the masculine domain of sport, with its noble pursuits of teamwork, competition and leadership. It is only in recent times that we are making headway in this area, but even now, you don't need to look far to see the inequities that still exist at the heart of almost every area of sport. For women, physical activity has always been about fitness and fitness has been intrinsically intertwined with diet culture. For generations, women's physical activity has been focused on burning calories. From jumping jacks to hula hooping, jazzercise to step aerobics, Zumba to spin classes – women have been sold a variety of solutions to the 'problem' of their bodies and encouraged to push themselves to their limits in pursuit of a smaller dress size.

This has led to many women having a troubled relationship with physical activity. For so long, it has been tied to feelings of shame, to the idea that they should always be doing more. So to tell women to get off the couch and get some exercise as a solution to their problems is always going to bring those feelings of shame and guilt to the surface – it will always sound to people as if they are being accused of laziness. There has been a moral component to exercise for so long that it is hard to hear it as a suggestion of something that might make you feel better – it will only ever sound like an accusation that you are neglecting your responsibilities.

Danielle Friedman, who wrote a history of women's exercise in the United States, found that while trends have emerged in women's fitness over the decades that have been empowering and confidence-building, the cloud of diet culture has hung over it all. 'At the same time as exercise became more accepted for women, it also became more expected of women,' she says. 'And with more opportunities, came increasingly greater pressures throughout the 20th century and then into the 21st century for women to meet an increasingly unrealistic beauty and body ideal.'[50]

As I find new ways to move my body without pushing myself too far or judging myself too harshly, it makes me realise the pure joy I am able to feel when I allow the cloud to dissipate. This is the kind of exercise I want to talk about. It is only when the shame and obligation are removed that genuine healing through exercise can begin, and I want to know how other people have found their path to this.

Emily is the first person I talk to about this topic – as a child and a teenager she found escape and refuge in sport when things were difficult at home. She loved how all-encompassing it was, how it didn't leave space to feel her other feelings. 'I would often get really angry and frustrated,' she tells me. 'I had all these awful feelings and emotions within myself, so sport was my outlet. I could run and make my feelings go away. I could do all these cool skills that took years of practice that focused on my anger and my anxiety. Every single feeling that I could have ever had was focused into sport, it very much was a physical way to recover for me.'

While it was not the only, or even the biggest, step in her recovery from a traumatic childhood, the energy it took up and the distraction it provided played the same role that work has played for other people. The ability to throw herself completely into an activity that allowed no space for difficult feelings that she wasn't ready to process was vital in the early stages of her healing. 'The more intense the game was, the better, because I pushed myself even harder,' she says. 'It literally would take all negative emotion away for months at a time. It was just weird. Even now when I go to the gym, it's the best release in the world.'

As a professional athlete, Sophie had work and exercise combined into one all-encompassing pursuit and – like Emily – she found space to breathe away from the feelings she wasn't yet ready to deal with. 'As soon as I got to training or a game, I was in the change room and my mind just switched off,' she says. 'Netball was all I was thinking about. I wasn't thinking about what I was going to do when I got home or anything like that. The distraction was really good – that was my chance to escape everything for a few hours.'

While playing sport did not necessarily help her in processing her emotions, Sophie found the care she needed to help with that in the chosen family she created within the team environment. The distraction of training was useful, but what mattered most was the people she surrounded herself with who were there for her when the feelings came rushing back. 'Reality would hit when I came off the court, and I'd just be thinking, I want to go home,' she says. 'It was hard to process the emotions, but I had the support of my teammates, and they'd often remind me that this is what Mum would want. They were right, my mum would have hated it if I sat at home and sulked, she would have wanted me to come to Sydney and play netball, and my teammates remind me that she's with me every step of the way.'

For Amy, the community around sport has been an important part of how she has healed. Her heart felt a little bit more whole again when elite netballers made the time to come out and support her fundraising initiative. 'The netball community has given so much to us,' she says. 'I think netball is always going to be a massive part of what the Tie Dye Project is all about.'

For Mel, exercise formed a later part of her recovery. While work and study were the areas of her life she used to throw herself in wholeheartedly to bury herself in distraction, recently sport and fitness have let her tread more gently along her path. 'My goal this year was to try and find some movement that made me feel good, not something that would feel like it was a chore,' she says. 'It definitely helps in clearing my mind and just making myself feel good for me and not for anyone else.'

Like me, Mel has found that introducing exercise slowly – and making sure it is something that genuinely brings her joy and doesn't add to her stress – has been important. Along the way she has found it has given her the space to grow into herself again. 'I've been going for walks and runs around my area, which has been lovely,' she says. 'And I've started playing tennis again, which has really got me feeling more like myself. I realised when it started happening that I haven't felt like this in a really long time. Knowing that I can go for a walk and it actually is something that can help me has been a nice change from exercise feeling like a chore.'

AJ has had a similar experience with exercise in the later stages of processing her trauma. Being active has been life-changing in this next stage of her recovery. 'We live quite near to the river, so any time I need to, I can just go for a walk,' she says. 'I can choose whether I want to be with my thoughts or listen to a podcast, but I'm in the fresh air and I think that has been a huge thing for me. I'm now in the routine of being active most days, which I think has been extremely helpful.'

While it's not always easy to get out the door on the more difficult days, when her feelings are overwhelming her, having the routine and momentum behind her has smoothed the path and given her confidence. 'I know when people are struggling mentally, that when someone says, "Go out and get some exercise", it can be easy to just say, "Fuck off, as if that's going to make a difference". But I know from myself and other people close to me that if you can just start doing it, it does make a difference. Having a routine helps and I definitely feel better and stronger.'

In her book, *This Ragged Grace: A Memoir of Recovery and Renewal*, Octavia Bright explores exercise as part of her own healing from a diagnosis of alcoholism and witnessing her father's increasing spiral into dementia. While initially she begins hiking as a distraction from her feelings, she finds a sense of herself along the way and the exercise itself becomes healing for her. 'It was as if I walked beyond something within myself, into a new state of calm that I hardly recognised as part of my own consciousness, a feeling of total wellbeing,' she says. 'On the path that day I first understood the difference between the kind of movement that's an escape from the self and the kind that's an encounter with it.'[51]

I feel like I understand better now that both of those forms of movement – the escape and the encounter – can be important parts of the recovery process for people who have been through trauma. While typically the escape comes earlier in the process and the encounter with one's self later, something else I have learned is that recovery is not linear. I suspect there will be times throughout the years that I need to dip back into escaping myself through movement, to run until all my thoughts are silenced and all I can focus on is the ache in my legs and the burn in my lungs.

It is a subject that Cheryl Strayed explores throughout her book *Wild: From Lost to Found on the Pacific Crest Trail*, which delves into the trauma she faces in the aftermath of her mother's death, her marriage breakdown and her subsequent issues with addiction. In the years that follow, she cycles through many different stages of recovering from trauma, but it is not until four years after her mother's death that she undertakes the monumental journey of hiking the Pacific Crest Trail and finds healing in the intensive nature of the physical activity. 'Uncertain as I was as I pushed forward, I felt right in my pushing, as if the effort itself meant something,' she writes. 'That perhaps being amidst the undesecrated beauty of the wilderness meant I too could be undesecrated, regardless of the regrettable things I'd done to others or myself or the regrettable things that had been done to me.'[52]

I first read *Wild* in 2017, when I had no concept of what it meant to have a life split by trauma. I remember finding it shocking, almost voyeuristic in the peek behind the curtain of trauma and recovery it gave me. I devoured it – racing my way through the pages and trying to get my head around all the parts of Strayed's life that had gone wrong and how she put herself back together. It seemed like a glimpse at a life I would never fully understand.

When I returned to the book after having cancer, it spoke to me in a different way. My experience of trauma is completely different from Strayed's and I still do not pretend to understand exactly what she went through. However, I now feel a deeper connection to her words and recognise the feelings of impulsivity and recklessness that burrow their way into the consciousness of a life touched by trauma. The need to both lose and find myself in isolation and exertion calls to me much more loudly than it did before.

I find myself overwhelmed by the wisdom I have collected and unsure of how to proceed with what I know

now. It seems naive that I once thought I could step back into my old patterns easily, that my relationship to physical activity would remain unchanged when so much else had shifted underneath and within me. I thought that I could erase my trauma through movement, but as Khoudari notes, that is not – and should not be – the aim. The comparison she draws to strength training is a fascinating one – when muscles are put under exertion during strength or resistance training sessions, this is actually referred to as 'muscle trauma'. The muscles suffer small amounts of damage, which disrupts their cells and activates satellite cells, which are drawn to the site of the trauma and begin stitching themselves to the muscle fibres to facilitate the healing process. This growth in cells in the muscles is what makes the muscles grow and become stronger – a process known as hypertrophy. Without this damage, they will never reach their full potential; while they remain whole and undamaged, they do not grow or become stronger.

It is a useful comparison and one I realise I need to come back to more often. Not just for the trauma experience as a whole, but specifically for my relationship to exercise after recovering from cancer. I remember the days after I ran a marathon – I had to take the next day off work because walking was so painful, and it was almost a week before I felt comfortable going up or down stairs.

If someone had asked me to run another marathon – or even a five-kilometre race – during that week, I would not have been able to do it with the same ease or flow that I had the week before. My muscles had been pushed to their limits, all their little cells damaged and disrupted, and I had to let them do the work of healing before I could try to push them again. During that time, I would not have even tried to push myself, or felt disappointed at my lack of ability. In that purely physical space, I understood that time and healing were required and I was content to be patient with my body.

It's not that I didn't think along these lines after cancer. I knew there would be ongoing physical effects and I thought that I had done what I needed to do in order to heal. I really thought I had given myself enough time, had gone at a slow enough pace, to return to where I was before. It wasn't only that the physical side effects of cancer treatment are much more extreme than the muscle trauma I suffered from running a marathon, it was also that those effects were stacked on top of the mental and emotional side effects that warped and stretched the recovery time. Emotional trauma and muscle trauma are not the same thing, even though they are sometimes connected. The comparison to muscle trauma works, but the timelines are different.

If I look at my recovery from cancer in the context of that week of post-marathon recovery, I am probably only on the third or fourth day. The extreme pain experienced on the first day is gone, I can make my way back to work, I can exercise gently. But I can't jump straight back to where I was before. I simply haven't given myself long enough to heal.

As frustrating as it can be at times, it can also be comforting to think about this elongated timeline. It gives me some hope that I will one day get back into a rhythm and find myself in movement again. It probably will not be that my muscles literally get stronger and I become a better athlete than I was before. After all, I am ageing every day and there is research to suggest that cancer treatments such as radiotherapy and chemotherapy accelerate the biological ageing process.[53] But that does not mean that I can't find momentum and rhythm in physical activity again. I might not ever make it back to that personal best time, but maybe I can find that same flow where it is not a matter of feeling every painful step along the path.

I love the idea that there are so many different ways that movement can help me heal. Even that five-kilometre run that hurt so much was valuable. Like Emily and Sophie found that sport allowed them to take their minds off what was happening in their personal lives, I certainly had no fears of cancer recurrence or anxieties about what the future may hold while I was grinding out that run. I was consumed by the immediate struggle, unable to think of anything at all except whether I could take my next step. As infuriating as it was to feel like my body was out of my control, the ability to shut my mind off and live completely in that moment is something worth appreciating. It was also something I experienced on the netball court – I was so annoyed at myself for missing so many goals or righteously angry at defenders who pushed and shoved to get their way that I had no mental space for more serious fears and worries.

It strikes me that pure distraction has been something I have continually discounted as part of the healing process. And yet I have heard time and again from people how important it was for them throughout different stages of their trauma. I have been so caught up in the idea that I have to really, deeply feel my feelings at every stage and worry when I don't do this that I haven't stopped to consider that some feelings are too overwhelming to experience in the moment. Distraction is a useful tool because it lets me put those overwhelming feelings away until I am ready to feel them. And while that is something I tend to associate with the early stages of trauma, there is still value in it now.

My understanding of the timeline I need to fully recover now takes in the emotional elements as well and I feel more willing to let myself get lost in distraction when I need to. Just because a certain amount of time has passed since my diagnosis, or my treatment ending, doesn't mean I need to feel a certain way. I have held this subconscious expectation of myself that I should adhere to a strict schedule of recovery that is based on almost nothing but my own idea that I should be better by now. And that I shouldn't need distraction as a tool. But I can now remind myself that although it feels like I'm moving slowly, I am going forward. I can't expect myself to run a marathon – physically or emotionally – when I am only on day three of my recovery week.

I also take a lot of heart from the way Amy speaks about community within sport and its importance for healing. Soon after finishing treatment, I wrote a story for *The Guardian* about the way the women's sport community rallied around me when I shared my diagnosis on social media. From professional athletes like Amy to other sports journalists, administrators and fans, I was cloaked in love from afar during a time when I felt incredibly alone due to Covid restrictions. Reading the story back now reminds me how lucky I am that so many people cared and that it all sprang from a simple shared interest in women's sport.

'Many of the people in this community I have never met,' I wrote at the time. 'We are spread across the country, across the world even, but we talk and share our stories almost every day. They are people I care deeply about and I was surprised and overjoyed to discover that they cared just as much about me.'[54]

As I start to move deeper into my recovery, I find AJ and Mel's approach to movement speaks to me more as well. This is the kind that Octavia Bright referred to as an 'encounter with the self', as opposed to the escape and distraction that I have found in running and netball. I definitely found this kind of movement with Ellen, when I learned to be patient and listen to my body. Like AJ and Mel, I also find it while walking.

In my running days, I found walking vaguely pointless unless I was actually trying to get somewhere. Walking for the sake of exercise felt too slow and unfulfilling. But during the pandemic, I found a sense of peace in walking that I was able to carry with me into cancer treatment. In both of those times of heightened emotion and uncertainty, walking felt purposeful. It gave me something to do and I could go with a friend and catch up, I could listen to a podcast or an audiobook or I could be with my thoughts. I could walk quickly or slowly, go long distances or short ones. It felt soothing, whichever way I did it. But until now, I haven't ever really thought about it as healing in itself.

When I have considered the idea of processing my trauma, I have pictured it coming in floods of tears or emotional breakthroughs during counselling. But what I understand now is that some of it has come through distraction, when my legs felt like lead and my lungs struggled to find air. Some of it has come through community, when people I had never met gathered around me in solidarity. And some of it has come through encountering myself over many thousands of steps and letting my thoughts wash over me. I know that I am only part of the way there and I will need to keep on moving, keep on processing, for a long time yet. But I finally feel like I am heading in the right direction.

CHAPTER NINE

Sunshine on a Rainy Day

'I'm feeling a beautiful sadness.'

A little over a year after my diagnosis, I sat at the Sydney Cricket Ground on Jane McGrath Day. Each year, the third day of the Sydney Test is dedicated to raising money for the McGrath Foundation and the stadium is swathed in pink. I had been planning to attend the year before, but I was too sick from chemo and not completely comfortable with the Covid risk to my compromised immune system. So I was looking forward to this day, but again my plans were thwarted – this time by rain. As I sat on the floor with Pia and my sister Lisa in a covered area of the Ladies' Stand while rain lashed down and prevented any cricket being played, I wondered if I would ever get any closure. I realised I had been hoping I would get some kind of meaning and understanding from this day – from seeing thousands of people come together and support breast cancer patients. Instead, I felt just as I always had – overwhelmed by the same numbness that left me with the impression that this was all happening to someone else.

It was the first time that I realised I had been waiting for a kind of lightning strike to shock me into action, some big, defining moment that would knock me over the head and make me suddenly understand how I should be living my life after going through the pain and sadness of cancer diagnosis and treatment. I thought I could watch Australian opening batter Usman Khawaja bring up his double century amid a sea of pink and all at once I would feel something that would lead me into creating my 'new normal'. And so as the clouds set up camp and the rain relentlessly marched on, I felt robbed of that moment. But even if there had been cricket played that day, would it have made a difference?

The idea of a 'new normal' is one that often arises after times of crisis. One of its earliest uses was following the First World War, when American inventor Henry Wise Wood pondered how the world could move on from such a catastrophic event. 'To consider the problems before us we must divide our epoch into three periods, that of war, that of transition, that of the new normal, which undoubtedly will supersede the old,' he wrote. 'The questions before us, therefore, are, broadly, two: How shall we pass from war to the new normal with the least jar, in the shortest time? In that respect should the new normal be shaped to differ from the old?'[55]

It is a question that has continued to arise in the decades since, with the September 11 terrorist attacks, the 2008 financial crisis and most recently the Covid pandemic prompting people to dust off the phrase and sprinkle it liberally across the media. That it has been so prominent is no surprise. To most people, normality represents stability, knowing with some level of certainty how things will turn out. In periods of great upheaval, most of us crave normality, even when we recognise that it may not look the same as it did before. So we rush toward the 'new normal', desperate to shape it, to understand how it may look and begin the process of getting used to it.

I have lived through a number of these new normals, and now understand that there is a difference between a world-changing event and a life-changing event. There is a limited amount I can control about what life looks like in a post-pandemic world, but after this deeply personal life-changing event, I need to decide how to remake myself, how I want to live after all this. Only I'm not sure where to start or what to do to make all this happen. At the heart of this is the feeling that I have lost my sense of self. I don't know how to create a new normal life when I don't truly know who I am anymore.

In *This Ragged Grace*, Octavia Bright discusses this disconnect between the selves in relation to her own alcoholism and her father's dementia. 'Traumatic experiences shatter the illusion of a coherent identity: they split your life into a before and an after,' she writes. 'Addiction and illness create a similar schism: between self and addict, between wellness and sickness, between person and patient. The time before the descent, and after.'[51]

From the moment I was diagnosed, I felt I split into multiple selves – the before person, who I know so intimately, but now feel worlds apart from. The during person, who endured all the pain while hiding behind a mask. And the after person, the one I can't quite get a grip on. She feels like she is floating just out of reach, and I need to understand her to be able to pin her down and let her step into me.

Until I do, I feel adrift from myself, a placeholder for a person. I keep marching on, doing everything I need to do, but I don't feel like I am experiencing any of it on a deeper level. It is not something I feel I have been able to resolve through counselling – I have struggled to get others who have not gone through it to understand. Instead, I feel I need the perspective of someone who has experienced their own schism as a result of trauma.

Mark

Something I love about my life after cancer are the conversations I never would have had before. I am very open about what I went through – some who have been on the receiving end of me telling them I had cancer within ten minutes of meeting them might say too open. I'm sure it makes some people uncomfortable or they think I just want attention (they would be right about that). But other times it leads people to reveal things about themselves that they otherwise wouldn't have.

While attending a youth camp for work about a year after completing treatment, I had a conversation with a teacher whose wife had died from cancer a few years previously. I doubt we would have come across the subject if it hadn't been for me oversharing, so I'm very glad I did. The way he spoke about his wife and her acceptance of her diagnosis and how they spent their final months together was incredibly beautiful and I felt so privileged to hear about it. His story will stay with me for a long time.

I contacted Mark after I returned home from the camp to find out more about his story. When I asked if I could write about it, his reply was 'Why not?' It is a perspective he has embraced over the past few years since his life changed dramatically.

Mark's story begins many years ago, when he was at university studying to become a teacher. It was there that he first met Lisa. 'I liked her straight away,' he tells me one evening, after riding his bike the twenty kilometres through bush tracks after a day at school to his quiet home overlooking the ocean. 'And then after a while, she started liking me back. We just became really good mates and then we fell in love when I was twenty and she was twenty-one, and we lived happily ever after. I'm sure everybody romanticises their relationships, but genuinely, we still felt the same way about each other thirty-three years later.'

So it was an incredible shock to the couple – both happily immersed in their jobs as teachers on the south coast of New South Wales – when some simple medical tests began to lead them down a more complex path. 'Lisa had been a bit unwell,' Mark says. 'An upset tummy and a little bit of pain, but nothing that I thought was particularly untoward. She was talking to the GP and they were looking at some dietary stuff, so they recommended a colonoscopy.'

Mark had been living with Crohn's disease, which required regular colonoscopies, so neither of them was particularly concerned. They travelled to Canberra for the procedure and had planned to stay the night and enjoy dinner at a nice restaurant afterward – it seemed like a good opportunity to have a night out together. But when Mark arrived to pick Lisa up and went to sit down in the waiting room, the receptionist told him the doctor had asked for him to go up to the room.

'At that point, my spidey senses just twigged a little bit,' he says. 'But I got up there and everything was great. Lisa was coming out of the anaesthetic and she was having a sandwich and everything was really pleasant. I noticed on the table there was a folder of images from a colonoscopy. I looked at one of the images and I don't know what a good colonoscopy looks like, but I remember thinking that it didn't look quite right.'

Before Mark had time to process those thoughts, the surgeon came to speak to them and he was not able to allay Mark's fears. 'I remember his words were, "The colonoscopy was very worrying",' Mark says. 'That was a real "oh fuck" moment, because even though my spidey senses were tingling, I never anticipated it was going to be like that.'

The surgeon went on to tell them that he had taken a biopsy and had sent it away for testing. While he was not able to confirm anything until the results arrived, he wanted to prepare them because he was fairly certain he knew what the news would be. 'He told us, "What I saw looks very much like bowel cancer and I'm almost certain it is",' Mark remembers. 'He then said to us, "In fact, if the biopsy came back and said it wasn't cancer, I'd send it away. Because I'm as close to certain of it being cancer as I can be." From that moment, nothing was ever going to be the same.'

It was as if the world had fallen out from under their feet. Up until this point, their life had been fairly close to idyllic. They had raised two happy, healthy daughters who were now in their twenties and were off having adventures of their own. Mark and Lisa were in their fifties, entering the twilights of their careers but still happy and fulfilled by their work. Mark was – and remains – the head of student wellbeing at a local high school, while Lisa was the principal at the town's primary school.

Mark felt shattered by the news. 'I remember having this feeling – and I reckon this is common – that stuff like this isn't meant to happen to me and my people,' he says. 'This happens to other people, but not me and my people. This isn't quite right.' Mark and Lisa walked out of the room feeling shell-shocked and unsure of how to proceed in the wake of this life-altering news. They walked to the car in stunned silence and drove to their accommodation. Their plans for a relaxing dinner out and a night in a nice hotel seemed from another life entirely.

'I don't think I spoke at all,' Marks says. 'I had no idea what to say. I wanted to be able to say something to make her feel better. I wanted to be able to say the right thing. But there was nothing I could think of that would make the situation better. We stopped and I turned the car off. I realised there was no need to bullshit, so I just said, "I want to say something, but I've got nothing. I don't know what to say and I'm just so sad".'

The two of them cried and hugged each other for a long time. Then, in the absence of a better idea – and because they needed to eat – they decided to keep their reservation and go out to dinner. 'We went to this beautiful Thai restaurant in Canberra, on the foreshore at Kingston, and it was really lovely,' he says. 'But we were just distraught, we were crying – really embarrassingly crying – but also we were holding hands. Later on, when our emotions had settled down a bit, we started wondering, what would someone who was watching us think was going on? We got a bit of a laugh out of that.'

From that point onward, they entered a downward spiral from which there seemed to be no escape. The surgeon had warned them that the tumour he suspected he had seen looked like a difficult one, in an area that would be hard to reach with surgery. 'From that first moment, we only ever got bad news,' Mark says. 'Basically, any fork in the road where things could get better or get worse, they got worse every time. Where the tumour was meant that surgery would be really problematic because he wouldn't be able to join it up after the bowel resection. It just kept going like that, bam, bam, bam, just bad news, bad news. It was fucked.'

Mark and Lisa had held off telling their daughters and parents as they knew as soon as they did, they would be dooming them to the same awful feelings they were plagued with. However, the time had now come to break the news. While everyone was devastated, they found some small joy as Mark and Lisa's oldest daughter returned home from overseas to be with her mother. As the news continued to get worse and Lisa began an aggressive chemotherapy regime, she pushed on at work. While Mark was initially not sure that was the right decision, he recognised that it was one Lisa needed to make herself.

'The whole time that she was sick, I was very aware that this wasn't happening to me, it was happening to Lisa,' he says. 'She was really proud of being a principal, it was a big part of her identity. If it was my choice, she would have retired straight away. But I knew she was going to feel a lot of grief around losing that part of her identity, so I had to let her come to that realisation herself. I'm really pleased that I didn't put pressure on her.'

For a while, Lisa found a way to continue – Mark would take her to chemotherapy in the morning, then drop her at school and she would sit in her office and work through the awful days that follow a session of having poison pumped into your veins. Mark and Lisa also took it as an opportunity to educate. They were both staunch realists and understood that the treatment was only going to buy them time. The cancer was aggressive and difficult to treat and there was only so long they could stave off the inevitable. 'Really early on, Lisa said, "This is the most important teaching I'll ever do",' Mark says. 'We knew she was dying, so we realised we could actually teach kids that bad things can happen – even the worst thing can happen, and it could still be okay.'

As Lisa was teaching primary school, she didn't want to overwhelm the children by providing too much detail, but she found age-appropriate ways to explain what was happening to her and the illness she was experiencing. Working with high school students, Mark was able to be more direct and upfront in his explanations. 'Lots of my kids had been Lisa's kids in primary school, so they knew her as well – it's a small town,' he says. 'I told them,

"Lisa's got cancer and it's not the sort of cancer you get better from. So I'm going to take time off to look after her. Lisa is not going to survive this cancer, so I'm going to be away from school a fair bit. I want you to know it's not because I don't care about you, it's not because I'm taking a holiday, it's for something really important." I wanted to teach them that we don't have to speak about death in metaphors, like "passing on" or "going to heaven"; we can talk about someone dying.'

Eventually, Lisa decided that she would retire – as much as she loved her work and would feel untethered from her identity, the combination of her illness and the treatment became too much to manage alongside a demanding job. She realised that if she retired, she would be able to access her superannuation, which would provide more financial freedom and the opportunity to do some of the things they had always wanted to do together. She was also able to access her life insurance before she died, at which point Mark says she 'tried to buy everything on the internet'.

'I loved that,' he laughs. 'I said yes to everything when she got sick except the puppy. Literally everything she wanted, I said, "Yes, darling, let's do it now." Then she said she wanted a puppy and I had to say no, because I didn't want to have the responsibility of looking after anything when I was by myself. I didn't know if I'd be able to do that. I would have loved her to have a puppy, but I felt like that would be more than I could handle.'

After her retirement, Lisa needed to relocate to Canberra for three months to have radiation treatment, which wasn't available in their small town. Mark knew that the time had come for him to take time off work as well and he travelled to Canberra with Lisa to be by her side throughout the treatment. Once she had completed radiation, they stayed in Canberra to meet with Lisa's doctor and review the results. As they had become accustomed to by now, it was not good news. The primary tumour had shrunk a little, but other tumours had emerged and the cancer had spread to Lisa's liver. As a last spark of hope, the doctors sent Lisa to Sydney to meet with a surgeon they believed may be able to help. Mark went along with her, although he wasn't sure that exploring the surgery route was the right thing to do.

'I had really mixed feelings about it because she had stage four metastatic terminal bowel cancer,' he says. 'She was going to die from it. It's possible that with surgery, she might live a little bit longer. But I had mixed feelings about her undergoing the trauma of major surgery and having a colostomy bag and for what? Another couple of months of life, with diminished quality. But I also wanted her to live for as long as she could. Both options were awful.'

However, the decision was taken out of their hands, as the surgeon in Sydney did not think surgery was viable in Lisa's case. The tumours were too big, too numerous and in difficult positions. He advised that if she underwent more treatment and the tumours shrank further, surgery could be a possibility. But deep in their hearts, they knew he was being kind and offering them one final thread of hope to cling to, rather than it being a real possibility.

Mark and Lisa were staying with Mark's dad and when they got back to his place, they crumpled to the couch and wept. The reality of reaching the end of the treatment road had hit and they were struck with waves of grief for the life they had dreamt of spending together. But only a short while later, Lisa sprang into action. 'She got up and said, "Right where's the computer?"' Mark says. 'She went and got her laptop and said, "Okay, we're going on holiday. I've got the passports. We're going tomorrow." My dad still talks about it – he describes it as the most courageous thing he's ever seen. That was Lisa all over – she knew we could stay sad, but fuck, what's the point? She decided that the best holiday she could find in the next hour was the Whitsundays. So by ten o'clock the next morning, we were on the plane to the Whitsundays.'

It wasn't long before Lisa's life began to wind down – her world became smaller and she stayed closer to home.

This happened to coincide with the pandemic and so with their daughters at home, the family allowed their world to become smaller too and they found joy and comfort in each other. 'I could work from home and that was perfect,' Mark says. 'For a long period of time, it was just the four of us at home and we were playing card games and listening to music and watching movies together. It was so special and so lovely. I felt guilty because we had friends whose businesses were going down the gurgler because of Covid and I knew there were people who were getting sick and dying. But I was thinking, I fucking love Covid. It was like we put a moat around our house and lifted the drawbridge up.'

Those months are seared in Mark's memory as some of the most special and poignant of his life. They knew how little time they had left as a family, so they made the most of each day and were able to have every conversation they had wanted to have. Most of all, it meant they left behind no regrets. 'It was just my beautiful family hanging out together and loving each other,' Mark says. 'And because we knew what was going on, we loved each other really hard. I feel so lucky that the girls got to spend time with Lisa, just one on one and both of them together. It was a unique set of circumstances.'

Lisa lived for eighteen months following her diagnosis and she made the decision early on that she wanted to die at home. In their small town, palliative care was mobile and it was conventional to allow people to spend their last moments in their homes. Under the care of two local GPs, Lisa slowly began to slip away from the world with her family by her side. 'She died with sun on her face and the nor'easter cooling her brow,' says Mark. 'We've got this lovely house on the hill overlooking the ocean. Her death was really beautiful. It was gentle and peaceful and lovely.'

While Mark took comfort in the fact that he had fulfilled Lisa's wishes and was full of love from the time they got to spend together, once Lisa had died, he felt an acute emptiness and more pain than he had been expecting. It was something he had been warned about by a colleague whose husband had died from cancer, but he was not ready to hear it at the time. 'My colleague said to me at one point, "Listen, I don't really want to say this to you, but this isn't the worst part. The worst part is going to be after Lisa dies." I felt a bit cranky with her and I remember thinking it was bullshit, how could it be worse than this? But it was because I was doing it by myself.'

While the past eighteen months had been about this awful thing happening to Lisa, once she was gone, the grief and loss were happening to Mark. He was no longer a partner who was supporting someone as they experienced something traumatic; this trauma was all his own.

When I speak to Mark, it has been two and a half years since Lisa's death and he is still finding the grief overwhelming at times. But he also realises that it is – at least in part – because he is holding himself back from moving on. The grief and the sadness connect him to Lisa, and he is afraid to lose that connection. 'It's really sad and lonely and I know, logically, it's not going to stay like this forever,' he says. 'We know that grief is always there, but it's not as raw forever. It's not as raw now as it was, but it's still pretty raw. I think if I was supporting someone else, I would have thought they'd be over it a lot more than I am by now. But I know part of me is also deliberately not moving past it because I want to be sad. I don't want to get over it.'

Mark has managed to find comfort in his grief and is able to frame it in joy and love. He speaks to me about the idea of his grief being a 'beautiful sadness', which is an idea that came from a surprising source – the cartoon South Park. 'I love that,' he says. 'I'm feeling a beautiful sadness. If I didn't have someone who I love so much, I wouldn't feel like I do now. The benefits of the joy and the love I have experienced for thirty-three years and will continue to, it's worth the sadness I've got. So that speaks to me, the idea of beautiful sadness.'

While Mark continues to hold that sadness close, he is also aware of not allowing himself to sink within it. A natural introvert, he knew that once Lisa died, he would need to consciously compel himself to leave the house and seek the company of others. While he enjoys his own company, he does not want to wallow in it. 'I've always been really happy on my own,' he says. 'Lisa has always been really social. If we were going out to parties, that would have been Lisa's doing and I'd be grumbling about it. I'd have fun when I get there, but that's not what I want to do. On a Friday night when I get home from work, I just want to hang out with Lisa and watch TV. So I've always known that I've got to be careful.'

Lisa knew this all too well and as part of her online shopping spree during her illness, she bought him a drone. It was as if she knew that Mark's deep bond with nature would be the string that pulled him from within himself and helped him reconnect with the world. Mark keeps the drone and his GoPro in a backpack and finds himself reaching for it when the darkness begins to descend. It is how he encourages himself to step out into the world and find the light. 'Whenever there's a camera in my pocket or my backpack, that is my reminder that there is beauty and joy everywhere, if you look for it,' he says. 'If I carry my camera with me, I see the sun going through the trees in a really beautiful way, so I stop and I take a photo of it and I get on my bike and go again. As a psychological tool, it has been powerful to remember that even on the worst day, if you just lift your eyes up above your shoes and have a look, you'll find beauty, you'll find joy, you'll find something to be grateful for.'

Work has been another outlet for Mark as he has tentatively re-emerged into the world. When he first returned to work only a month after Lisa's death, he initially found it too much to cope with and realised he had rushed back. 'I thought I'd go back to school because I didn't know what else to do,' he says. 'I went back for day one, term one. That was really hard. I got to the end of term three, and I had to go to my boss, who's one of my best mates, and tell him I needed a break. I was so worried that there would be a day when I wasn't on top of my game and I'd miss something and it could end with a kid attempting suicide. I would never forgive myself for that.'

During his time off, Mark considered his future. Once Lisa had received her superannuation and life insurance, they had been able to pay off the house, leaving Mark without a mortgage and able to finish working completely if he so desired. Over the months, he fell into a rhythm of surfing every morning, heading home to read for a few hours, then taking an afternoon bike ride with his trusty backpack and cameras in tow. He also sought out psychological help, realising that he had been advising students to set up mental health care plans and speak to psychologists for many years and it was time for him to take his own advice.

It was a gentle and peaceful period of his life and for a time, Mark considered that it may be the way he would go on forever. He couldn't see himself reaching a point where he would be able to give his job the energy, focus and passion it needed. But whenever he thought about giving up the job, an ache in him made itself known and he could not allow himself to fully commit to a life without this meaningful and important work. Late in the term, Mark's boss called and asked him about his plans for the following year. He told him that although he didn't want to put any pressure on him, they were writing the timetable and he really felt like he needed Mark to return. It was exactly what Mark needed to hear. 'When he called, I heard that I still had a contribution to make,' Mark says. 'It meant that he really valued my contribution and the school was better, the kids were better, if I was there.'

In the years since, Mark has come to understand what it is about the job that clung on so tightly to his heart. His job offers him a way to make a difference and to do good in the world, and this is inherently tied to his sense of self. 'I've realised that a big part of who I am, who I want to be, is that I really want to be proud of myself,' he says.

'It's a level of arrogance where I think part of who I am is doing good, is making the world a better place. If I wasn't doing that in some way, then I would lose a sense of who I was.'

While he recognised that there were other ways for him to make a difference in the world, he also knew that he was very good at his job. It was a well-worn path for him, but that only increased its significance, as he could return to it and immediately be of value. 'If you asked me to fix a car, I'd have no idea,' he says. 'I have no skills whatsoever, I'm less than useless. But I'm really good at this. I'm really good at finding the right thing to say at the right time. It's just that – without being a wanker – I think empathy is something that comes easier to me than to other people.'

And so he returned to school and settled back into the familiar cadence of the bells, classes and conversations. While it wasn't the same as it was before Lisa died, he found new ways to talk and relate to his students and slowly re-immersed himself in this life. 'Sometimes kids come in and they're devastated because their Instagram post didn't get many likes, or their friend has left them on read,' he says. 'I've always had this ability to listen without judgement, even if what they tell me might sound to someone else like it doesn't matter, it matters to them in that moment, so it matters. It's always come really naturally. But I've found

I've got to work harder at it now. Everything's a bit harder since Lisa died; my emotional reserves aren't quite as deep now.'

Mark's life is quieter and smaller than it was before, but there are little things that reach through his ongoing grief and keep him tethered to the world. While solitude was part of his process early on, he has now started to let more people in. 'I started going to sleep in the bush two nights a week,' he says. 'I'd light a fire and sit there by myself and sleep under the stars. I've always loved being in nature, so that gave me great comfort. Then one day I was talking about going to do it and one of my mates said, "I'll come with you." It's evolved now where there's a group of seven of us and every Monday night, we camp in the bush together. We're all in bed by 8:30 pm and we're up at six o'clock to get to work. We don't have a beer or anything, we just light a fire and get together. It started with them looking after me, but now it's a lovely group of mates who sit around a campfire every Monday night and just enjoy each other's company.'

As to where his life goes from here, Mark remains unsure. He has spent the last few years gathering these puzzle pieces to assemble a life after Lisa, but he has not yet found out the way they all fit together. 'I've got no idea what the rest of my life is going to look like,' he says.

'I haven't cracked the code, I'm not sure how to live a happy life now. The train is on the tracks, the house is tidy, I'm looking after my girls, I'm cooking dinner every night and I'm going to work. To someone outside looking in, it would look like I'm doing fine. I'm getting everything done. But I've got no idea how I'm going to lead a happy, productive life. I've got faith in my ability to work it out at some point, but I'm not there yet.'

In the meantime, he is content to discover the answers slowly, to keep finding those pieces and gradually assembling them. One thing he is sure of is that he will continue to carry Lisa with him. His life will always be intertwined with hers.

Our conversation is long and meandering, wandering off in unexpected directions. Both of us have long given up on leading linear lives and it feels like our conversation reflects this. Down one such conversational laneway, Mark tells me about his old habit of referring to himself as 'Freddy', a nickname he shared with his dad and his brother from their cricket playing days. When he was particularly happy with a dinner he had cooked or a task he had done well around the house, he would say to himself 'Good one, Freddy' as he admired his work, something that made Lisa and his daughters laugh and roll their eyes in equal measures.

'When Lisa was sick, we would write little love letters to each other every day,' he says. 'She started signing off "Good one, Freddy" which was our little joke. A couple of months after she died, I was looking through some of her things and I found one of these notes. I'm not a tattoo guy, but a couple of months ago, I got a tattoo in her handwriting that says, "Good one, Freddy" with a couple of kisses on my forearm. On a rough day, she's there with me saying hang in there, keep going. But part of it is also that if any other woman looked at me and thought I seemed nice, they're going to see that I belong to Lisa.'

As we reach the end of our phone call, Mark is removing his roast vegetables from the oven, nearly ready to sit down to dinner after a quiet whisper of 'Good one Freddy' to himself. He may not have his life completely worked out, but he is doing a good job treading water until he – in his words – 'cracks the code'. The past few years have provided a steep learning curve and he shares some of the wisdom it has left him with.

'I'm not scared of anything anymore, because whatever happens, I know that it won't overwhelm me,' he says. 'I have absolute faith in myself that on the worst day, I can handle it. The worst thing that would happen for me would be if one of my girls got sick. And I'd fucking hate it. But I'd handle it. I know now that I can deal with anything.'

* * *

Although both Mark's and my experiences are entangled with cancer, on the surface, there is not much else that links them. But the way he speaks about his life is so deeply relatable and I recognise the identity split in the way he recounts his experiences. He too had a self that existed before Lisa's diagnosis, a self that supported her through her illness and a self who lives now, tinged with grief in the aftermath of her death. I consider many times throughout these conversations I am having just how lucky I am that my cancer was treatable, that we caught it early enough. Without those strokes of pure luck, this would have become Shaun and Pia's story, and the idea of the full burden of trauma falling on them is almost unthinkable.

I take a lot from the way Mark talks about his 'life after' as a work in progress. Unlike that lightning strike of realisation that I have subconsciously been looking and waiting for, his patient way of marking time until he 'cracks the code' seems more realistic, less urgent. Where I have felt this treading water in between my life as a cancer patient and the 'new normal' is something I need to overcome, Mark seems to understand it better as a key part of the process. Perhaps this is a fourth self we are experiencing – an in-between person who keeps this body safe until the after person is ready to take over. Just because this person doesn't have it all figured out yet doesn't mean they are less important, or their contribution to the whole is less meaningful than that of the other selves.

I also come to understand the role that grief plays in my story. Although it is a drop in the ocean compared to the immense grief that Mark has been faced with, the grief of losing my former self is not something that I have consciously grappled with. I have recognised the identity schism, but I have not fully understood why it troubles me so much and from which depths the sadness about it has been dragged.

When Mark speaks about how a part of him is deliberately not moving on from his grief, that the sadness he feels is his last remaining connection with Lisa, there is a resonance. I too can sense something inside of me that is holding me back from moving on. There is a fear camped out in a little corner of my consciousness that by fully grasping the after person and allowing her to step into me, I will be letting go of the before person – I will never be her again. And while I know deep down that nothing can bring her back, I cannot shake the feeling that if I maintain this connection to her, by refusing to let my new normal envelop me, I can somehow become her again.

Cheryl Strayed writes in her 'Dear Sugar' advice column about a disconnection from her former self that she discovered while transcribing her old journals. 'I felt rattled and kind of sick for the rest of the day, as if I'd been visited by a phantom who both buoyed and scared the bejesus out of me,' she writes. 'And the weirdest thing of all is that phantom was me! Did I even know her anymore? Where did the woman who'd written those words go? How did she become me?'[56]

Even without a cancer diagnosis, I would eventually have become removed from my old self. I know logically that I was not the same person before I was diagnosed at thirty-six as I was when I was nineteen. I would always have looked back on fragments of my past and wondered at how much I had changed and perhaps felt some sadness at losing parts of myself. But this particular feeling of the self being so suddenly torn apart has not given me time to slowly let go of the person I was and absorb the new person bit by bit. I feel resentful that it has been forced upon me, that she has been ripped from me so completely.

In re-reading the work of CS Lewis, Hilary Mantel started to understand the way all kinds of loss – no matter how insignificant it may seem compared to the loss of a loved one – mirrors the process of grief in the body. 'Disbelief is followed by numbness, numbness by distraction, despair, exhaustion,' she writes. 'Your former life still seems to exist, but you can't get back to it; there is a glimpse in dreams of those peacock lawns and fountains, but you're fenced out and each morning you wake up to the loss over again.'[57]

It is a sentiment that resonates – feeling trapped by loss and grief for the ghost of a life that continued on with the chimerical version of myself who did not get sick. I am not sure how to process all this – they were feelings I didn't even realise I was having until I sat down to examine them more closely. But I am sure that the sadness I'm holding on to as a way to keep me connected with my former self is playing a role in keeping me inside this placeholder version of myself.

Former Reuters journalist Dean Yates was ambushed by trauma symptoms when his years of reporting on traumatic events such as the 2002 Bali bombings caught up with him and he had to begin the hard work of processing his feelings. But even when he began to understand what was happening, he discovered that he was only just scratching the surface, intellectualising the experiences and not feeling them.

'There is no "aha" moment – it's not a straight line where you all of a sudden start to feel well,' he told *The Guardian*. 'When you do work at healing from trauma ... you can find a new normal – a higher level of functioning, greater levels of empathy. And that can be found in the journey of recovery itself.'[58]

I think now that I am better equipped to do this work of healing and find my new self. I am no longer looking for shortcuts, no longer hoping an Usman Khawaja sweep shot will awaken me into a new life. My 'after' self is not hiding behind swathes of pink in a sports stadium, fully formed, ready to jump out and envelop me in her arms. She is much more likely to be found in little bits and pieces. I catch a tiny glimpse of her in my conversation with Mark and more little flickers in the other conversations I have had. I have found a twinkle of her in Pia's hugs, a glimmer in Shaun's laugh and a sparkle in my mum's care.

Rather than wait for a fully realised person to appear, I can catch these little pieces as they fall and begin the process of stitching together my new self. I can decide who I want to be and manoeuvre these pieces as I collect them, trying them out in different places as I discover how they fit together as a whole. I can start to let go of some of the sadness and grief for my former life by consciously being more curious about my new self and trying to get to know her. I can appreciate that I am made up of different selves and not feel that I have to move through one into the next, but maybe hold some together for a while.

I am considering this one day while reading *Anne of Green Gables* to Pia – a book that my grandmother adored and I had never been able to get through as a child, as desperate as I was to love it too. I have taken so much joy in reading it with Pia, as she and Anne are very much 'kindred spirits' as Anne would no doubt put it if they met. I was not expecting to find wisdom in those pages, but it comes to me one morning as we read the book before school. 'There's such a lot of different Annes in me,' I read. 'I sometimes think that's why I'm such a troublesome person. If I was just the one Anne, it would be ever so much more comfortable, but then it wouldn't be half so interesting.'[59] It's been a transformative way to think about my selves and the different aspects of me they bring to life. While I haven't yet 'cracked the code' of how to live the life I want, for now, it is enough to realise that I can stop feeling impatient with this placeholder person who is occupying my body and be kinder to her. She is as much a part of me as my other selves.

CHAPTER TEN

I Am Here

It is two years to the day since my diagnosis and I am sitting in the radiology waiting room. Everything is pink. Being diagnosed with breast cancer during breast cancer awareness month is very confronting at times. I'm here because the scar tissue in my breast has a similar appearance to a tumour in the ultrasound. For the past year, my surgeon and the radiologist have been going back and forth, monitoring it and trying to decide what to do. Eventually, they have decided that we will bite the bullet and do a biopsy. The report from the radiologist has the words 'a biopsy is suggested to exclude local recurrence'. Reading it feels like being struck in the face, like a horror movie coming to life. That word 'recurrence' feels so loaded and I don't know how to cope.

Naturally, when I tell people what is happening, I talk it down. I feign irritation with the process, I act as if I'm being forced into the biopsy, that I would have just left it if it was up to me. 'It's annoying, but we've got to do it, so we've got the results to show the radiologists when they raise it in future,' I tell my husband, my mum, my boss. 'I'll just get this done and then I don't have to think about it anymore.' But on the inside, I'm not annoyed. I would have chosen to do this, even if my surgeon had said it was unnecessary. I'm too scared it could be something serious to let it just sit inside me, unknown. One night as I'm falling asleep, I catch myself thinking, *When I have chemo this time, I need to remember to ask if I should have a port.*

When I have chemo.

This time.

I wish my insides matched my breezy exterior, but I think I have already gone back into survival mode. Pessimism may be unhelpful in some situations, but it feels necessary here, like I have to brace myself for the impact that I feel certain must be coming. I squeeze my eyes shut through the biopsy, making sure I have no chance of seeing the big device that makes the terrifying clicking sound as it is pushed into my breast four times to collect the sliver of the mass they can see on the ultrasound. It is ten days before I get the results and for all that time, I feel like I am in a heightened state, constantly alert for the moment when it all falls apart. The logical voice within me – the voice that speaks on the outside too when I reassure my friends and family – says that my doctor would have called me sooner if it was bad news. They would not have waited ten days for the scheduled phone call to break the news.

But until my phone rings at 8 am on that Monday morning, I don't – and I can't – believe it.

'Hi, I'm just calling with the results of the biopsy you had the other week,' the doctor greets me when I answer. 'It was all consistent with scar tissue, so no problems there. So let's organise your scans for next year.'

It is over in an instant – the worry, the plans for how I would survive a recurrence. I expect to feel a deep relief, maybe even an outpouring of emotion, but I don't. I think about that *Hunger Games* moment I had envisioned as being my reaction to the news of a recurrence and in that moment, I know that it would not have played out that way. I am still braced, still in survival mode. I am not sure I am capable of that level of feeling, even to the worst news. I am relieved that I do not have to go back and relive that trauma, but it is a surface level relief, something that feels more akin to an item ticked off a to do list than a life-changing moment. It is frustrating to feel this way, to get this far and still not have all the answers. I have always been an impatient person and this rush to feel normal again is not unexpected. But alongside the frustration and the rush sits acceptance – it is just a small amount, but it is growing larger every day and its voice is growing louder, calmly telling me that it is okay to be in this state, to occupy the in between for however long it takes.

If I'm being honest with myself, I expected to have more answers by the time I got to the end of this book. I envisioned spinning it all together into an expertly woven tapestry, with all the loose ends tied up and a beautiful vision of the future looking back at me. Instead, I feel like I have a jumble of questions, more even than when I began. In answering some of the questions I had at the beginning, more have arisen and I am left wondering when and how I could ever answer them all.

I am pondering this one day, walking along in the spring sunshine, when a sentence in an audiobook I am listening to jumps out at me. 'It's not enough to survive, you've got to live.'[60] The book is Abi Morgan's *This is Not a Pity Memoir* and the story is deeply grounded in trauma. Morgan's partner collapsed one day and spent months in hospital in an induced coma, sustaining brain damage that caused him to not remember her on waking. During these difficult times, Morgan herself was diagnosed with breast cancer and had to embark on treatment while also trying to help her husband come back to himself. The line sends a jolt through me – all this time, I had been so determined to discover whether there is more to my life after trauma than survival and this line offers me a moment of clarity. I have survived cancer and all its associated trauma, but the emptiness and numbness I feel is because I have not yet worked out how to live. Once I press my concerns into that shape, I feel things start to click. The thought raises more questions than it answers, but at the same time, it provides the framework I need to start to understand what comes next.

I begin with contemplating my fear of recurrence, and the awful idea of not even surviving. My conversation with Greg was heavy with emotion and it contained so much wisdom. His fight is for survival – he is doing everything he can to be there for his family, to keep on going until he finds a treatment that works. But although he has been forced into a focus on survival, it is not limiting because he is already living.

From Greg, I learned the power of hope, of living for each day in spite of fear for what the future holds. Greg's own future is less certain than mine and he feels the fear about this acutely, but rather than try to conquer it or push it away, he allocates it to its own little compartment. It is always there, ready for him to examine it and understand better how to live with it, but on days where it feels overwhelming, he can close the lid and focus on the joys of the day.

I remember once interviewing Australian netball great Sharelle McMahon who spoke about courage, telling me that it wasn't about 'being fearless, because everyone has fears ... Courage is about having those fears and jumping anyway.'[61] Greg's courage is profound. He has found a way to go on in the world in the face of incredible hardship and deep, unknowable fear. While I originally set out to find a way to eliminate – or at least minimise – my fear of recurrence, I have learned from listening to Greg that that is not necessary or even ideal. I will always live with the fear of my cancer returning, but rather than let it consume me, I can compartmentalise it and assign it to its proper place. I don't like feeling afraid – it is an uncomfortable feeling, and thinking about living with permanent fear puts me on edge – but it is a feeling that penetrates the numbness and makes me feel alive. Fearing death is a reminder that I want to live, want to experience growing old and meeting all the different versions of myself I will become in the future. It will always be a part of me, but I don't need to let it be my defining feature. Living with fear is not the same as living *in* fear.

Likewise, my anxieties about parenting will never leave me. Even when Pia is an adult, with a life of her own, I have no doubt I will continue to worry about her. About whether I did enough for her, about the invisible marks my illness and its associated trauma have left on her. From my conversation with Emily, I learned that those worries never truly disappear, but that over time, they can become more manageable. There is a passage in Bridie Jabour's *Trivial Grievances* about parenting that seared itself in my brain:

> I thought it was a love that would become more manageable over time, but a woman told me she feels the same way about her adult children that she did when they were toddlers. It seems impossible. If this is true, how does my father ever stop hugging me? How does my mother survive months without seeing me? How do my parents just go to work, go to the shops, see their friends and have a life, knowing their children are somewhere else, possibly making bad decisions? Drinking? Probably with people who wouldn't throw themselves in front of a car to protect them? How do you exist knowing they are boiling kettles by themselves thousands of kilometres away, and anything

could happen with a boiling kettle? (I will have to ask them one day when I remember to call.)[28]

As Pia has grown older, she has begun collecting small acts of independence and each one fills me with pride and breaks my heart at the same time. The first day she walked the last part of the way to school on her own, I couldn't truly relax until I saw her when I got home from work that evening. Parenting is about constantly letting go, and it is hard and joyful at the same time. Whether or not I had experienced this trauma, I would have had these worries about Pia and how the decisions we have made as parents have affected her and shaped who she becomes. Trauma has complicated these feelings, as I feel in a hurry to see her grow up at the same time as wanting to hold her close to me. But from Emily, I have taken a genuine understanding of the importance of letting kids have a childhood. As much as I feel the need to participate in all these milestones and rush toward them, Pia's life is not about me. If I should one day get a recurrence and end up missing some of these important moments, I will have to make my peace with that. Pushing Pia into adulthood before she is ready will not make that time any easier for either of us; it will only add another layer of difficulty to her life. Hearing Emily's story about the ongoing effects of a childhood ripped from her by trauma reiterates the importance of making sure that as many children as possible can experience the joy and freedom of being young. I can't protect Pia from every misfortune, but I can protect the freedom of her childhood and let these little independence milestones happen slowly, at her pace.

My understanding of friendship has shifted through reflections on my conversations with Heather. Not only has it shifted my perspectives on the way I make and maintain friendships, it has also highlighted the importance of those support systems outside family. Trauma has so many impacts and it truly takes a village to get everything you need during those times. Friendship is not a relationship our society often takes seriously – certainly not as seriously as family and romantic relationships – but when life falls apart, the importance of having this extended community suddenly becomes very clear. While trauma makes that need very acute, friendship is necessary for everyone: the Irish Longitudinal Study on Ageing found that it even correlates with a longer life and better health outcomes.[62]

Taking the time to reflect on my friendships has forced me to reconsider facets of myself and to appreciate my friends even more than I already did. Friendship looks different to everyone and those who I choose to hold close were there to weather the storm with me – whether or not they were physically by my side. I can see now how vital this support system was – and continues to be – in helping me process what I have been through. Every walk, every TV episode watched together, every invitation to dinner, every meme sent in the group chat made me feel a little bit more myself and a little bit more able to face the world. Through my friends I have learned how to experience joy again, even if it doesn't quite feel real all the time. Through them, my understanding of myself has shifted and this new person – the 'after' person who I am slowly becoming – is one who has fierce friendships, full of love and loyalty.

Through my conversation with Mel, I have become gentler with myself about the way I used work as a distraction during my illness. There is still a part of me that grieves for the time lost and wonders whether I would have been better if I had been able to shut down at least some of that distraction and focus on myself. But discovering and understanding the usefulness of distraction – particularly in the early stages of trauma – has made me feel better about my decisions. I have been able to draw back a little from my need for productivity and recognise now that the actual process of work and occupying my brain in that specific manner was more important than needing to achieve or find validation in my work. Mel's contentment with her life and the peace she has made with herself in the wake of her trauma are good indicators of the purpose distraction can serve, and how she was able to slowly process her trauma in a way that was meaningful and not overwhelming.

With time and the fresh start that has come from settling into a new workplace, I have been able to find what is important to me in this new life. I have settled on the idea of wanting to make a difference through my work, no matter how small that difference is. It is something I feel can guide me forward and keep me grounded. The feeling of losing control of myself during my illness will stay with me for a long time – perhaps forever – and a sense of purpose through work is something I feel that can be an anchor to stop me drifting back into that loss of control, whatever may come. While it does not provide any certainty about the future, it does make me feel more able to deal with the uncertainty.

Purpose is also something I want to bring into my personal life. The stories of Amy, Sophie and Molly strengthened my resolve to make a difference in the world. Through these young people, I feel I have a better sense of how advocacy can guide me and the meaning that can be found in a life that takes me in such a direction. While I have struggled with some of the ways breast cancer is portrayed, and the commercialisation and sexualisation of the disease, I think I need to not just sit back and bemoan this, but step forward and try to do something about it. The widening of my scope of advocacy means I can also provide support in other spaces and find causes that align with my values.

But the reality is that as much coverage as breast cancer gets, people are still dying. It may receive more than its fair share of attention, but a significant amount of that attention does not bring any money in; rather, the focus is on the much more vague 'awareness'. And while the treatments have comparatively good success rates in a lot of cases, the drugs themselves are far from ideal. One of the main chemotherapy drugs for breast cancer is doxorubicin, colloquially referred to as the 'red devil', the use of which dates back to the 1960s.[63] It is commonly combined with cyclophosphamide, which is a derivative of mustard gas. These treatments have remained in use because they often work at ridding the body of cancer, but words cannot do justice to the awful experience of living through them.

There is undoubtedly more to be done to find treatments for breast cancer that not only work towards zero deaths, but also provide quality of life for people going through it. Advocacy for this kind of research is best articulated by those who have experienced the current treatments, so I can see that I do have a role to play in moving this cause forward. However, the understanding I have taken from listening and learning – particularly from Amy – means that I can cast a wider net and give myself space to breathe outside of a cause that can sometimes feel suffocating.

The ongoing ways both my illness and the trauma surrounding it will continue to touch my life are not so easily reconciled. It is going to take a lot of work to not feel resentful of all the ways my life and my body feel different after cancer and treatment. AJ's thoughtful message of gratitude has stayed with me and, little by little, has buried itself into my consciousness. I have learned that being grateful does not mean embarking on a course of toxic positivity and that it is okay that some days I can't summon gratitude. Slowly, I am letting myself feel grateful for my life in a way that does not stop me from mourning what I lost. It's hard and the two states don't always sit side-by-side comfortably but, with time, I feel sure I will get there.

AJ has been a great inspiration to me. She has come through immense trauma and shaped a life that is all her own on the other side. As she herself notes, this takes a certain amount of privilege; it is not something that everyone is able to do. But this does not take away from the work AJ has done to carve out a life for herself and the incredible love and care she is capable of. Giving back to the world is something she too has found powerful – as well as the purpose she finds in paid work, AJ also spends a lot of her free time volunteering, which is something I connect with as I often joke that I am a chronic volunteer. This personality trait is one I inherited from my dad and one which I am sure Shaun would love me to leave behind, especially when my volunteering is so chronic that he often gets roped in as well. But it is helpful to me to think about it slightly differently in the wake of trauma. It makes me realise that not every aspect of making a difference needs to change the world. Doing a little bit of admin work as a team manager that makes it easier for more young girls to participate in sport has its own importance and power, and I can acknowledge these small acts as part of my recovery, and how I have begun to process my emotions and make sense of myself. Framing my experiences this way has been another small step in finding my new self.

Coming to terms with my body and its changed abilities has been immensely challenging, but the process of comparing my recovery to the way muscles break down and reform after exercise has helped me make better sense of the timeline I am working with. Over the months of considering this, I have learned to be kinder to myself and gentler with my body. I have not yet overcome my tendency to judge my body and wish I could shrink it, but I feel that

I'm on the path toward it. The different ways that exercise can form part of the healing process after trauma continue to sit with me, and I have begun cautiously exploring these different modes of movement, allowing my body to slip in and out of encounters and escapes as I go.

As I start to get into a busy part of the year, my days and nights fill up with clashing commitments, most involving ferrying Pia around to her different sports and activities, but also with work and social engagements. A few weeks into this bustling period, I feel a gnawing emptiness, a discomfort I can't quite name or pin down. It takes me a little while to realise that I have not made time to exercise, and my mind and body are feeling this lack. It's different to the way I have felt in the past – when I was a dedicated runner, it was a restlessness, an itch in my bones that pushed me back out to capture that rhythmic addiction I found on the footpaths. This feeling is not as intense; it is a quieter unease, one I could have easily ignored or chalked up to something else if I had not taken the time to examine it. It clicks then, the importance of movement in my recovery, in finding my new self. She is not the same person as that relentless runner, but she too wants to move, needs to move. It is the first time I have an understanding of her that is more than just a glimpse.

In Victoria Hannan's *Marshmallow*, the central incident of the novel is the sudden death of a child – a trauma that cracks and refracts throughout a group of the child's parents and their friends. The child's father, reflecting on the plans he had made before they were all destroyed, expressed a thought that stuck with me: 'He hadn't known then what he knew now: that the future didn't exist.'[64] It has been an interesting way to reframe looking at the future – as something imagined, nothing more than fantasy. No matter how much planning and preparation is done, there is no way to control the future, no guarantee that it will play out the way we have envisaged. The future I had imagined before I was diagnosed disintegrated and slipped away as soon as I heard those words, 'You have cancer.' But that is true of all futures: they are unreal, mythological beings.

My conversation with Mark is where I truly start to feel at peace with this idea and understand it fully. Mark too had plans for a future that flew from his grasp when Lisa was diagnosed and eventually died. He has had to regather himself and start again, moving toward a future he had never planned for, never thought possible. But the plans he makes – and I make – now are different. Once you have experienced trauma snatching the future from your hands and reminding you that it is all in your imagination, you can never again step toward it with the same energy. And so we approach plans in a way that is more cautious, not daring to make them too detailed or too distant, lest they be taken from us again. It is something we are both learning to overcome, this extreme caution. Tied so closely as it is to my fear of recurrence, I don't think I will ever leave it behind completely. But I can plan for the future in different ways, when I recognise that it is imaginary and with the knowledge I will be okay if it all falls apart. I can dream, wish and wonder all the while figuring out my new self and, as Mark would say, learning to 'crack the code'.

When I try to find the words to describe why I needed to write this book to figure all this out, it is Cheryl Strayed's *Wild* that again makes it clear. 'I had problems a therapist couldn't solve; grief that no man in a room could ameliorate,' she writes. While I – and most people I have spoken to – have relied on the services of psychologists, I understand now that what I have experienced is bigger than that room I sat in to share my fears and worries. I could never fit it all in, could never explain it all. I needed to – I still need to – find other ways to make it smaller so that I can carry it with me without being weighed down. But after all this talking and listening and writing, I feel closer to it. The enormity of it doesn't scare me so much anymore.

That complete emotional breakdown may still be coming, and if it does, I have confidence in my ability to handle it, whether it flows out as a trickle or a flood.

I don't have all the answers – I may even have fewer answers than I started with – but turning experiences into stories has helped me make sense of them. Stories have always been the way I have understood the world and laying mine out has helped me make peace with myself.

* * *

It is late at night and I am reading to Pia. It's way past her bedtime – she has become a master at playing on my love of books, of reading with her, to stretch out this nightly ritual where we read to each other snuggled under the blankets of my bed, usually with our cat, Rory, in between us. Rory finds her way into this position so regularly that I start to suspect she likes to hear the stories too.

We are up late because we are trying to finish *Anne of Green Gables*. I like to think my nan is there too, standing at the end of the bed, delighted I have finally made it to the end of this book. In the final chapter, we encounter one of Anne's many monologues. She is talking about her change of plans after the death of one of her guardians and the illness of the other.

> When I left Queen's, my future seemed to stretch out before me in a straight road, I thought I could see along it for many a milestone. Now there is a bend in it. I don't know what lies around that bend, but I'm going to believe the best does. It has a fascination of its own, that bend, Marilla. I wonder how the road beyond it goes – what there is of green glory and soft, chequered light and shadows – what new landscapes – what new beauties – what curves and hills and valleys farther on.[59]

I pause after reading it, feeling those words soak into my consciousness. Pia pushes herself up into a sitting position.

'Can you read that bit again?' she asks. I do and we both sit in silence for a few moments as we take it in.

'I think that's the best quote in the whole book,' Pia says.

'Yeah, I think so too,' I tell her. 'What do you like about it?'

'I can just imagine it exactly the way she says it, with the hills and the grass and everything,' she says. 'I like thinking about the future that way, like it's somewhere we can walk, but we don't know exactly where it goes yet.'

It's a really lovely moment, just being with her and sharing our love of stories. We finish it and talk about our favourite parts and whether Anne should have forgiven Gilbert Blythe earlier for calling her 'Carrots'.

'I can't wait to start our next book,' Pia says as she finally goes off to bed.

'Me either,' I say. 'Let's start thinking about what to read next and when we should read the next book in the Anne series.'

It's a very small plan for the future, but something about it feels revolutionary. It comes without caution or fear – it's just a natural step forward, toward that bend in the road. I don't know exactly what lies ahead and where that bend will take me. But suddenly, I have a feeling about that path that I didn't before. Wherever it leads, it goes on.

References

1. 'Trauma.' Australian Psychological Society. Accessed October 27, 2023. https://psychology.org.au/for-the-public/psychology-topics/trauma.
2. Sunderland, Matthew, Natacha Carragher, Cath Chapman, Katherine Mills, Maree Teesson, Emma Lockwood, David Forbes and Tim Slade. 2016. 'The shared and specific relationships between exposure to potentially traumatic events and transdiagnostic dimensions of psychopathology.' *Journal of Anxiety Disorders* 28 (March): 102–109.
3. Center for Substance Abuse Treatment (US). Trauma-Informed Care in Behavioral Health Services. Rockville (MD): Substance Abuse and Mental Health Services Administration (US); 2014. (Treatment Improvement Protocol (TIP) Series, No. 57.) Appendix C, Historical Account of Trauma. https://www.ncbi.nlm.nih.gov/books/NBK207202/
4. Young, Robin, and Karyn Miller-Medzon. 2023. 'Psychiatrist Judith Herman on trauma, justice for survivors and her passion for social justice.' *WBUR*, May 16, 2023. https://www.wbur.org/hereandnow/2023/05/16/judith-herman-abuse-survivors.
5. Atkinson, Meera. 2021. 'More than half of Australians will experience trauma, most before they turn 17. We need to

talk about it.' *The Conversation*, April 29, 2021. https://theconversation.com/more-than-half-of-australians-will-experience-trauma-most-before-they-turn-17-we-need-to-talk-about-it-159801.

6. Salter, Michael, Martin Dorahy, and Warwick Middleton. 2017. 'Dissociative identity disorder exists and is the result of childhood trauma.' *The Conversation*, October 4, 2017. https://theconversation.com/dissociative-identity-disorder-exists-and-is-the-result-of-childhood-trauma-85076.
7. 'Acute Stress Disorder – PTSD: National Center for PTSD.' National Center for PTSD. Accessed October 13, 2023. https://www.ptsd.va.gov/understand/related/acute_stress.asp.
8. Paddock, Catharine. 2019. 'New PTSD blood test could aid prevention and treatment.' *Medical News Today*, March 14, 2019. https://www.medicalnewstoday.com/articles/324709.
9. Klimova, Aleksandra, Isabella A. Breukelaar, Richard A. Bryant, and Mayuresh S. Korgaonkar. 2023. 'A comparison of the functional connectome in mild traumatic brain injury and post-traumatic stress disorder.' *Human Brain Mapping* 44, no. 2 (February): 813–824.
10. Wimalawansa, Sunil. 2013. Post-Traumatic stress disorder: An under-diagnosed and under-treated entity. Comprehensive Research Journal of Medicine and Medical Science (CRJMMS). 1. 1–12.
11. Duek O, Seidemann R, Pietrzak RH, Harpaz-Rotem I. 2023. Distinguishing emotional numbing symptoms of posttraumatic stress disorder from major depressive disorder. Journal of Affective Disorders. 324 (1): 294–299, https://doi.org/10.1016/j.jad.2022.12.105.
12. Lawrenz, Lori, and Janina Fisher. 2021. 'Trauma-Related Dissociation: Symptoms, Treatment, Coping, and More.' Psych Central. https://psychcentral.com/pro/coping-with-trauma-through-dissociation.
13. Chan, Caryn Mei H., Chong Guan Ng, Nur Aishah Taib, Lei Hum Wee, Edward Krupat, and Fremonta Meyer. 2018.

'Course and predictors of post-traumatic stress disorder in a cohort of psychologically distressed patients with cancer: A 4-year follow-up study.' *Cancer* 124 (2): 406–416. 0008-543X.

14. Barton, Adriana. 2018. 'For patients fighting cancer, PTSD is one more battle.' *The Globe and Mail*, January 31, 2018. https://www.theglobeandmail.com/life/health-and-fitness/health/for-patients-fighting-cancer-ptsd-is-one-more-battle/article37813930/.
15. Brown, Lauren C., Amy R. Murphy, Chloe S. Lalonde, Preeti D. Subhedar, Andrew H. Miller, and Jennifer S. Stevens. 2020. 'Posttraumatic Stress Disorder and Breast Cancer: Risk Factors and the Role of Inflammation and Endocrine Function.' *Cancer* 126, no. 14 (July): 3181–3191. 10.1002/cncr.32934.
16. Atkinson, Judy. 2002. *Trauma Trails, Recreating Song Lines: The Transgenerational Effects of Trauma in Indigenous Australia*. Spinifex Press.
17. Bahr, Jessica. 2023. 'What is intergenerational trauma and why is Jacinta Price being criticised?' *SBS*, September 15, 2023. https://www.sbs.com.au/news/article/what-is-intergenerational-trauma-and-why-is-jacinta-price-being-criticised/dif30u8aj.
18. Bar-Haim, Yair, Murray B. Stein, Richard A. Bryant, Paul D. Bilese, Ariel B. Yehuda, Morten L. Kringelbach, Sonia Jain, et al. 2021. 'Intrusive Traumatic Reexperiencing: Pathognomonic of the Psychological Response to Traumatic Stress.' *American Journal of Psychiatry* 178, no. 2 (February): 119–122.
19. 'Symptoms – Post-traumatic stress disorder.' NHS. Accessed October 19, 2023. https://www.nhs.uk/mental-health/conditions/post-traumatic-stress-disorder-ptsd/symptoms/.
20. Lee, Bri. 2018. *Eggshell Skull*. Allen & Unwin.
21. Delaney, Rob. 2022. *A Heart That Works*. Hodder & Stoughton.

22. 'Online Calculator Helps Predict Risk of Hormone-Receptor-Positive Breast Cancer Returning Elsewhere in the Body.' 2018. Breastcancer.org. https://www.breastcancer.org/research-news/online-tool-predicts-hr-pos-recurrence-risk
23. Liu, Jia. 2021. 'Novel Clinician-Lead Intervention to Address Fear of Cancer Recurrence in Breast Cancer Survivors.' *JCO Oncol Pract.* 17 (6): e774–e784. https://pubmed.ncbi.nlm.nih.gov/33571035/
24. Tovey, Josephine. 2023. 'Cancer is the pits at any age. But rates are rising in young people like me, and we don't fully know why | Josephine Tovey.' *The Guardian*, August 2, 2023. https://www.theguardian.com/society/2023/aug/03/cancer-is-the-pits-at-any-age-but-rates-are-rising-in-young-people-like-me-and-we-dont-fully-know-why
25. Rushton, Gina. 2022. *The Most Important Job in the World.* Pan Macmillan Australia.
26. 'What is Epigenetics? The Answer to the Nature vs. Nurture Debate.' n.d. Center on the Developing Child at Harvard University. Accessed September 17, 2023. https://developingchild.harvard.edu/resources/what-is-epigenetics-and-how-does-it-relate-to-child-development/
27. Haydar, Amani. 2021. *The Mother Wound.* Pan Macmillan Australia Pty, Limited.
28. Jabour, Bridie. 2021. *Trivial Grievances: On the Contradictions, Myths and Misery of Your 30s.* HarperCollins Publishers Australia.
29. Petersen, Anne H. 2019. 'How Millennials Became The Burnout Generation.' *BuzzFeed News*, January 5, 2019. https://www.buzzfeednews.com/article/annehelenpetersen/millennials-burnout-generation-debt-work
30. Kreider, Tim. 2012. 'The 'Busy' Trap – The New York Times.' *The New York Times Web Archive*, June 30, 2012. https://archive.nytimes.com/opinionator.blogs.nytimes.com/2012/06/30/the-busy-trap/

31. Carleton, R. N. 2015. 'PTSD personality subtypes in women exposed to intimate-partner violence.' *Psychological Trauma: Theory, Research, Practice, and Policy* 7 (2): 154–161.
32. Chouliara PhD, Z., T. Karatzias PhD, and A. Gullone BSc(Hons). 2014. 'Recovering from childhood sexual abuse: a theoretical framework for practice and research.' *Journal of Psychiatric and Mental Health Nursing* 21 (1): 69–78.
33. Colley, James. 2023. 'Becoming a father changed my perspective on everything, including dad rock.' *The Sydney Morning Herald*, August 31, 2023. https://www.smh.com.au/lifestyle/life-and-relationships/becoming-a-father-changed-my-perspective-on-everything-including-dad-rock-20230830-p5e0mp.html.
34. Infusino, Katherine. 2014. 'From Survivor to Advocate: The Ther ocate: The Therapeutic Benefits of Public apeutic Benefits of Public Disclosure.' *College of Education Theses and Dissertations* 63, no. 1 (March): 1–85. 1.
35. Mullins, Saxon. 2023. 'Sexual Violence Advocate Saxon Mullins On The Power Of Community In The Face Of Lifelong Pain.' *marie claire Australia*, March 7, 2023. https://www.marieclaire.com.au/survivor-saxon-mullins-on-the-power-of-community.
36. Maurice, Megan. 2023. 'Wish you were here: A year of grief, love, struggle and success.' *UNSW Newsroom*, November 3, 2023. https://news.unsw.edu.au/en/sophie-fawns--year-of-grief--love--struggle-and-success
37. Boyer, Anne. 2019. *The Undying: A Meditation on Modern Illness*. Penguin Books Limited.
38. Coopdizzle. 2016 'October is the best and worst month for me and my stage 4 sisters.' Facebook, October 2 2016. https://www.facebook.com/CoopdizzleBC/photos/a.1417707771815714/1762931640626657/?type=3
39. 'Pink Ribbon Marketing Culture.' n.d. Breast Cancer Action. Accessed September 11, 2023. https://www.bcaction.org/pink-ribbon-marketing-culture/#

40. Roper, Caitlin. 2022. 'Saving women, not 'boobies': The sexualisation of breast cancer.' Collective Shout. https://www.collectiveshout.org/sexualisation_of_breast_cancer
41. Wechsler PT, DPT, PhD, Stephen, Janet Kneiss PT, DPT, PhD, Benjamin Adams PT, DPT and Lisa J. Wood Magee PhD, RN, FAAN. 2022. 'Persistent Cancer-Related Fatigue After Breast Cancer Treatment Predicts Postural Sway and Postexertional Changes in Sit-to-Stand Strategy.' *Rehabilitation Oncology* 40, no. 4 (October): 162–171. 10.1097/01.REO.0000000000000308.
42. Silverstein, Amy. 2023. 'Opinion | My Transplanted Heart and I Will Die Soon.' *The New York Times*, April 18, 2023. https://www.nytimes.com/2023/04/18/opinion/heart-transplant-donor.html?smid=tw-share
43. Sarner, Moya. 2018. 'Is gratitude the secret of happiness? I spent a month finding out.' *The Guardian*, October 23, 2018. https://www.theguardian.com/lifeandstyle/2018/oct/23/is-gratitude-secret-of-happiness-i-spent-month-finding-out
44. Sirois, Fuschia M., and Alex M. Wood. 2017. 'Gratitude uniquely predicts lower depression in chronic illness populations: A longitudinal study of inflammatory bowel disease and arthritis.' *Health Psychology* 36 (2): 122–132. https://doi.org/10.1037/hea0000436.
45. Chun, Sanghee, and Youngkhill Lee. 2013. I am just thankful': the experience of gratitude following traumatic spinal cord injury.' *Disability and Rehabilitation* 35 (1): 11–19. 10.3109/09638288.2012.687026.
46. 'Body Positive Gym Sydney.' | Haven Wellness. Accessed October 24, 2023. https://www.havenwellness.com.au/.
47. Khoudari, Laura. 2021. *Lifting Heavy Things: Healing Trauma One Rep at a Time*. Wonderwell.
48. Rosenbaum, Simon, C. Sherrington, and A. Tiedemann. 2014. 'Exercise augmentation compared with usual care for post-traumatic stress disorder: a randomized

controlled trial.' *Acta Psychiatrica Scandinavica* 131, no. 5 (December): 350–359. https://doi.org/10.1111/acps.12371.

49. Pebole, Michelle, Chelsea Singleton, Katherine Hall, Stephen Petruzzello, Reginald Alston and Robyn Gobin. 2022. 'Exercise preferences among women survivors of sexual violence by PTSD and physical activity level: Implications and recommendations for trauma-informed practice.' *Mental Health and Physical Activity* 23 (October). https://doi.org/10.1016/j.mhpa.2022.100470.
50. Friedman, Danielle. 2022. 'The complicated history of women's fitness | On Point.' WBUR, April 18, 2022. https://www.wbur.org/onpoint/2022/04/18/the-secret-history-of-womens-fitness.
51. Bright, Octavia. 2023. *This Ragged Grace: A Memoir of Recovery and Renewal.* Canongate Books.
52. Strayed, Cheryl. 2014. *Wild: A Journey from Lost to Found.* Atlantic Books.
53. Wang, Shuo, Anna Prizment, Bharat Thyagarajan, and Anne Blaes. 2021. 'Cancer Treatment-Induced Accelerated Aging in Cancer Survivors: Biology and Assessment.' *Cancers (Basel)* 13, no. 3 (January): 427. 10.3390/cancers13030427.
54. Maurice, Megan. 2022. 'Here if you need': how warmth of women's sport community helped me through cancer.' *The Guardian*, July 21, 2022. https://www.theguardian.com/sport/2022/jul/22/here-if-you-need-how-warmth-of-womens-sport-community-helped-me-through-cancer.
55. Wood, Henry A.W. 1918. 'Beware!' *Bulletin – National Electric Light Association* 5: 604–605.
56. Strayed, Cheryl. 2023. 'What You Know Changes – Cheryl Strayed's Dear Sugar.' Cheryl Strayed's Dear Sugar. https://cherylstrayed.substack.com/p/what-you-know-changes.
57. Mantel, Hilary. 2014. 'Hilary Mantel on grief.' *The Guardian*, December 27, 2014. https://www.theguardian.com/books/2014/dec/27/hilary-mantel-rereading-cs-lewis-a-grief-observed.

58. Marsh, Walter. 2023. 'Detachment was considered a strength': how a war correspondent's calling created a trauma timebomb.' *The Guardian*, July 2, 2023. https://www.theguardian.com/society/2023/jul/02/detachment-was-considered-a-strength-how-a-war-correspondents-calling-created-a-trauma-timebomb.
59. Montgomery, Lucy M. 1987. *Anne of Green Gables*. Angus & Robertson.
60. Morgan, Abi. 2022. *This is Not a Pity Memoir*. John Murray Press.
61. Sinclair, Jennifer C., and Megan Maurice. 2016. *Shine: The Making of the Australian Netball Diamonds*. Finch Publishing.
62. 'The Irish Longitudinal Study on Ageing (TILDA) – Trinity College Dublin.' 2022. The Irish Longitudinal Study on Ageing (TILDA) – Trinity College Dublin. https://tilda.tcd.ie/news-events/2022/2204-tilda-waystolive-longer/.
63. 'Doxorubicin – StatPearls.' 2023. NCBI. https://www.ncbi.nlm.nih.gov/books/NBK459232/.
64. Hannan, Victoria. 2022. *Marshmallow*. Hachette Australia.

Acknowledgements

This book was written on the lands of the Wangal and Bidjigal peoples of the Eora and Dharug nations. I pay my respects to their Elders past and present. Sovereignty was never ceded and this always was and always will be Aboriginal land.

To the team at Hachette – thank you so much for your work and support of me. I am truly grateful for the opportunities I have been given and the way you have worked to make this book all that it can be. To Sophie Hamley – it has been such a delight to work with you over two books and you are such an inspiration to me. Chrysoula Aiello – thank you for the huge amount of effort you put in, your passion and your support. To Libby Turner and Emily Stewart – thanks for your eagle-eyed editing, which has made this book so much better. To the wider Hachette team, including Louise Stark,

Vanessa Radnidge and Fiona Hazard, thank you for your confidence in me and helping me put this story out into the world. And to my early readers, Helen and Stuart Maurice and Shaun Hardy, who read chapters and gave feedback when I wasn't sure I knew what I was doing – thank you for helping me build these stories into a book.

To my interviewees – Greg, Emily, Heather, Mel, Amy, Molly, Sophie, AJ and Mark – thank you for trusting me with your stories, it has been an honour to be able to share them. I wish you hadn't had to experience trauma, but I am so inspired and awestruck by how you have managed it.

To the managers and colleagues who supported me through illness and writing this book – Monica Melki, Peter Harrison, Helen Bryson, Mark Wright, Roger Carter and David Maxwell from UNSW and Karen Jones, Samantha Feyzeny and Steve Norris from the Office of Sport – without all of you, I would not have been able to tell this story. Thank you for your support through the hardest times of my life and beyond.

To my two co-authors from my previous books, Jenny Sinclair and Alex Blackwell – thank you for making me an author and giving me the confidence and skill I needed to write my own story.

To my editors, Mike Hytner, Emma Kemp and Jo Khan, everything you have done has made me a better writer and

I will always be grateful for your feedback and tweaks that have made my writing more readable. And to two of my teachers who made me feel like a writer before I was one, Scot Frazer and Helen Breen, your belief in me has brought me where I am today.

To my cancer comrades – Jo Tovey, Greg Harris, Na'ama Carlin, Kylie Mulligan and Vickie Saye – I never would have got through cancer as well as I did without you all. Thank you for keeping me company in the trenches and understanding when no one else could.

To my friends who were there throughout my treatment and beyond – Ana, Adam and Azucena; Alex, Lynsey and Edie; Kirsty; Jenn, Craig and Bec; Leanne and Amy; Alice, Taj, David, Claire and Frieda; and the Summer Hill Lakers Netball Club and Summer Hill Cricket Club – thank you all for being there for me and giving me somewhere safe to land.

To my family – Mum, Dad, Lisa, Matt, Bailey and Alana – for all your love, support and letting me play the cancer card whenever I felt like it and for continuing to care even after it was all over. It means the world to me. And to my in-laws – Pam, Ken, Louise, Mark, Luke, Ashley, Katrina, Rhys, Annabelle and Harry – thank you for welcoming me into your family all those years ago and always making me feel loved.

To Shaun and Pia – without you, this story would never have existed. Your love makes my work and my life possible. Thank you for everything, I love you both to the ends of the universe (and all the multiverses Pia, because I know you'll ask).

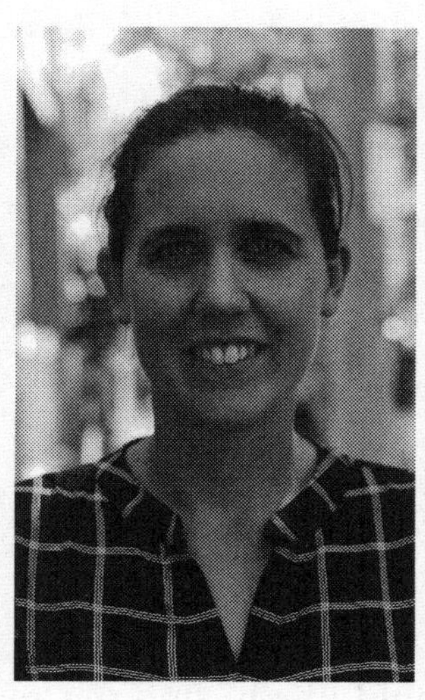

Megan Maurice is an award-winning journalist and the co-author of *Shine: The Making of the Australian Netball Diamonds* and of *Fair Game* by Alex Blackwell (Hachette, 2022). Her journalism has been published widely and she is a regular contributor to *The Guardian*, with a particular focus on issues of equity, diversity and inclusion. She lives in Sydney with her family.

hachette AUSTRALIA